Living Chi

THE ANCIENT CHINESE WAY TO BRING LIFE ENERGY AND HARMONY INTO YOUR LIFE

Living

THE ANCIENT CHINESE WAY TO BRING LIFE ENERGY AND HARMONY INTO YOUR LIFE

Chi

Gary Khor

Tuttle Publishing
Boston • Rutland, Vermont • Tokyo

This edition published in 2001 by Tuttle Publishing, an imprint of Periplus Editions (HK) Ltd., with editorial offices at 153 Milk Street, Boston, Massachusetts, 02109. Originally published in Australia in 1999 by Simon & Schuster (Australia) Pty Limited.

Library of Congress Cataloging-in-Publication Data

Khor, Gary, 1947-
    Living chi : the ancient Chinese way to bring life energy and harmony into your life /
by Gary Khor.
        p. cm.
    Includes bibliographical references and index.
    ISBN 0-8048-3274-9 (pbk.)
        1. Qi (Chinese philosophy) 2. Mind and body--China. I. Title: Ancient Chinese way
to bring life energy and harmony into your life. II. Title.

B127.C49 K49 2001
613--dc21   00-052772

Distributed by

North America
Tuttle Publishing
Distribution Center
Airport Industrial Park
364 Innovation Drive
North Clarendon, VT 05759-9436
Tel: (802) 773-8930
Tel: (800) 526-2778
Fax: (802) 773-6993

Japan
Tuttle Publishing
RK Building, 2nd Floor
2-13-10 Shimo-Meguro,
Meguro-Ku
Tokyo 153 0064
Tel: (03) 5437-0171
Fax: (03) 5437-0755

Asia Pacific
Berkeley Books Pte Ltd
5 Little Road #08-01
Singapore 536983
Tel: (65) 280-3320
Fax: (65) 280-6290

06 05 04 03 02 01   9 8 7 6 5 4 3 2 1

Printed in the United States of America

Contents

Introduction

Chi is one of the most profound concepts in the Eastern world, a concept that permeates the whole of Chinese culture. References to chi are found in subjects as diverse as medicine, philosophy, calligraphy, painting, bonsai, martial arts, and Feng Shui, to name but a few.

But what is chi?

On a cosmic scale, chi is described as the vital breath or energy that animates the universe. It is a sea of energy that permeates everything from the smallest atom to the largest galaxy. This concept has been present in Chinese thinking for at least 2,500 years. The ancient Taoists were very familiar with the concept, and now modern discoveries in both medicine and physics tend to support their theories.

On a more personal level, the Chinese believe an unobstructed flow of chi through the body to be essential for our physical and mental well-being. Stress is regarded as being one of the major inhibitors to the free flow of chi. It is appropriate, therefore, that the first chapter of this book examines relaxation in depth and the traditional Chinese approach to achieving it.

As you progress through the ensuing chapters, you will discover how chi affects just about all aspects of your life, and how you can harness and maximize this "cosmic energy" to improve your health and lifestyle. Topics covered include breathing, massage, meditation, diet, Feng Shui, and exercise.

I hope you will find this book to be both informative and helpful. I encourage you not only to read and understand *Living Chi*, but to set the chi concept to the test by putting into practice the principles and techniques explained in this book.

A number of people have contributed in various ways to the writing of this book and my thanks go to them all. In particular, I would like to thank David Walker for his assistance in the research and development of material, Sheila Boston for preparation of the manuscript, Gayna Murphy for the design and layout of the book, Gwenda Bate and June Williams for proofreading the manuscript, and last, but by no means least, Rod Ferguson for curriculum research and development.

GARY KHOR

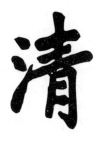

Chapter One

Relaxation

INITIATING WHAT WESTERN SCIENCE calls the "relaxation response" is the fundamental principle underlying the health benefits of Shibashi, Tai Chi, Qigong (Chi Kung), or other similar Chinese health exercise systems. If one cannot initiate the "relaxation response," one not only cannot perform these arts correctly but the major health benefits of the exercise systems will be lost.

Since relaxation is such a crucial component of Chinese health exercise systems, it is interesting that Chinese concepts of relaxation are in close accordance with the latest discoveries and thinking of Western science.

While the "relaxation response" can be initiated through the performance of various relaxation techniques with little knowledge of what relaxation is and how it works, quicker and better results can be obtained if the process is understood. The theory outlined in this section can be applied to all Chinese health exercise systems.

RELAXATION OR STRESS REDUCTION?

Relaxation or stress reduction — on what should we focus? Today, we mainly hear of relaxation only as the opposite of stress — as though relaxation is simply the absence of stress rather than a state in itself. There is endless talk of excess stress and the dangers it poses to our health, relationships, and productivity. (Latest estimates are that stress underlies

85 percent of sickness and disease suffered.) We are so focused on the negatives of stress, we are becoming "stressed out" over stress!

Most people understand enough about psychology to know that if they focus on words with negative associations they may well bring about the very conditions they seek to avoid. Successful athletes do not visualize failure and how to avoid it — they visualize success and what it feels like. It makes sense, then, that in our thinking we should be focused not on what excessive *stress* feels like and how such adverse effects can be reduced, but on the positive state of relaxation.

Unfortunately, many of us have such stressful existences that not only can we not remember what it was like to be relaxed but our concepts of *relaxation* are a little vague.

There was a tale told by one instructor of a student practicing Tai Chi in a park. The arm movements were all done with his shoulders raised (which is a sure indicator of stress and tension in the shoulder area, a common problem today). Wanting to be helpful, the instructor suggested that he try relaxing his shoulders. "But I am relaxed!" responded the student indignantly.

Telling someone to relax when he or she does not even know what relaxation is, let alone what it feels like or how the state can be achieved, is more likely to have a stressful than a relaxing result. As you read on, you will learn not only why relaxation is important but ways of initiating relaxation and to check if a little more relaxation can be achieved. First, let's look at exactly what is meant by "relaxation."

UNDERSTANDING RELAXATION

Tell the average person to relax and he or she will probably go and lie down. The meaning of relaxation is taken to be, "do nothing" or, more specifically, have your muscles do nothing. This is the "jellyfish on the beach" approach to relaxation — collapsing into a shapeless blob! Over time, this approach is about as healthy for the human body as it is for the poor stranded jellyfish.

This is particularly so today, when our lifestyles tend to be too sedentary to start with. We spend far too much time sitting in front of desks, at steering wheels, televisions, and computers, for our relaxation to be of a sedentary nature.

When our lifestyle involves little movement and we stop moving muscles, our muscle tissue begins to disintegrate. Without the pumping, massaging effect of the muscles, the circulation of blood, particularly in the venous system, becomes slow and congested; the heart has less blood to circulate but it must be circulated at a higher pressure, in order to force it through the congested tissue. Over time, as toxins accumulate and less oxygen and nutrients reach the internal organs, they start to fail and malfunction.

The body's defensive system relies on the circulation of the lymph fluid through the lymphatic system. This circulation has no pump and depends on movement to provide a massaging effect. As we reduce the amount of body movement, the body is less able to ward off pathogens.

As the body ceases to perform energetic activities, the level of mental energy falls off rather than builds up. We become less able to cope and more prone to depression; our sense of well-being dissipates and our relationships with others wither and die.

As an old Chinese saying goes, "it is the unused door hinge that gets eaten by worms." This is certainly not what we set out to achieve when relaxing!

Alternating a mainly sedentary lifestyle with a burst of violent exercise one hour a week only makes matters worse. It's like leaving your car in the garage for a month, then taking it out on a racetrack to loosen things up. The only reward you are likely to get is a blown engine.

When we seek relaxation we are trying to let go of unwanted stresses and tensions; we are seeking balance and harmony, not only at the physical level but at the mental and emotional level. One cannot even relax one's muscles if the mind is in a tense and agitated state, as the mental tension flows out and tightens them. When we think "relaxation" we must think holistically; we must achieve the optimum relaxation, not only for all the body's physical and metabolic systems but for all mental and emotional aspects as well.

If we think of a person who engages in no physical, mental, or emotional activity, "relaxed" is not the first word that springs to mind in describing such a state. Living involves doing, yet, according to some modern psychology, stress arises when the results of something we are doing do not match the predicted outcome, or do not match our expectations.

Such statements lend themselves to the argument that we should therefore do nothing, since that way our expectations cannot be disappointed and stress cannot arise. This is the type of relaxation we can get from experiences like float tanks; they can provide a great boost to health and a change in stress levels but, in essence, they are defeatist. It is said that you cannot relax in the real world, that you must withdraw from it. Is this true? Is there no technique of doing things that does not cause us to be stressed when our expectations are disappointed?

What we are seeking is a process of doing things, while not actually doing, while not being concerned with outcomes; for dealing with things as they are, rather than as we believe they should be. The Chinese have a name for such an approach — *Wu Wei*.

Wu Wei—the way to relaxed doing

Wu Wei is a difficult term to translate exactly. "Doing without doing" and "acting in accordance with nature" capture only some of the nuances. The *"Tao Teh Ching"* of Lao Tse, one of the greatest Chinese philosophers, expresses more of the flavor:

- Less and less effort is used, until things arrange themselves.
- Harmonious action retains control; exertion upsets the balance.

Other analogies used to express the essence of *Wu Wei* are:

- The woodworker cuts with the grain, not against it.
- If you get caught in a rip you do not exhaust yourself swimming against the current, neither do you let yourself get swept out to sea; you try to use the current, rather than defeat it.

One of the most illuminating stories is that of the Chinese butcher who as a novice wears out a knife every three months. As he becomes skilled at his trade, the knife lasts a year or longer; when he has mastered his art, the knife lasts ten years, although the butcher is cutting more meat than ever.

Wu Wei is, in fact, a whole philosophical approach to life, with many other implications which it is not appropriate to discuss here. What we are interested in is the application of this approach to relaxation.

It is easy to see that if we grit our teeth, summon all of our determination and say, "I am *going* to *relax*!!!" then it is doubtful we will. Concern over whether we are relaxed, together with agitation over signs that we are not, is hardly going to move us closer to relaxation. In fact, it seems the one thing we need, to be able to relax, is to be relaxed. No wonder people have so many problems achieving relaxation.

This is where the *Wu Wei* approach comes into its own. You do not *try* to relax, you simply perform those techniques which lead to relaxation (to be discussed later); you do not worry about whether you have *become* relaxed (to have expectations about relaxation), rather you simply have total awareness of what you are doing and feeling when you perform the relaxation technique. Don't concern yourself about what you *should* feel, or about what others feel, or that some unplanned event or noise might disturb "your" relaxation. Just be there; experience the moment — this is the *Wu Wei* path to relaxation.

There is the analogy of the Master Oriental Archer, who would draw and fire his bow in a relaxed, flowing movement, almost liquid in appearance. Startling levels of accuracy were achieved, but often the Master Archer would not even bother to establish whether he had hit his target, being totally dispassionate about the result. All that could be done had been done before the arrow left the bow; the focus was on the technique of firing the arrow. Of course, if the archer could focus on the technique of firing without being disturbed about whether he would be successful or not, the result was much more likely to be successful.

In relaxation, as in all things, decide what your objective is. Select techniques of action that should achieve your objective, then forget the objective and focus on experiencing the techniques. Of course, you periodically seek feedback to assure yourself you have selected the right techniques, but during the "doing," enjoy and be aware only of the doing.

RELAXATION AND ENJOYMENT

If you are going to carry out an activity without concerning yourself with its outcome, the activity itself should be intrinsically enjoyable. If it is not, stress will arise because you are spending your time doing something that is not gratifying. The activity must also be sufficiently demanding to challenge you (or boredom will set in) but not beyond your abilities (or frustration will set in).

Such intrinsically enjoyable activities are what have been referred to as "autoletic activities." Autoletic activities are those engaged in because they are rewarding now.

Studies of activities that were greatly enjoyed by those who performed them have showed the participants felt they were doing something new and challenging.

Autoletic activities have also been called "flow activities." Flow activities arise when there is such total involvement that action follows upon action, with no conscious intervention. There is a merging of action and awareness that eliminates the internal critic who asks "Am I performing well?" and "Am I getting it right?"

This, again, sounds very like a *Wu Wei* approach. Not only is there a dispassionate approach to the outcome, there is a passionate approach to the actual doing. The ancient Taoist is said to have meditated, not to improve himself, but because the process was enjoyable.

Truly enjoyable experiences improve one physically, mentally, emotionally, and spiritually. Experiences which cause us physical, mental, emotional, and spiritual pain are not truly enjoyable. (Who was it who persuaded us that eating, drinking, exercising, working, and accumulating money and possessions to excess, taking drugs, shocking our senses, and outraging our sense of moral rightness was enjoyable?) That which is truly enjoyable is also uplifting. How do you know when you have done enough of any activity? It ceases to be enjoyable!

This is a long way from the "no pain, no gain" slogan (which is perhaps better characterized as "short-term gains, for long-term pains"). Pain is a stressor; it is a warning that something is wrong, and should have no place in any sensible, long-term health program.

"Flow experiences" are common for people practicing Chinese health exercise systems, for the following reasons. The movements are connected into flowing sequences. The basic movement patterns can be grasped and performed by persons of all ages and health conditions, so frustration is not felt. There is, however, such depth of theory and knowledge connected to the movements that they provide a lifetime of experience, so boredom does not set in. Also, because of the focus they require, the movements lead to greater internal awareness.

DYNAMIC RELAXATION

We have defined relaxation as when the body, mind, and emotions are in harmony with each other. Let us in the future refer to this as "dynamic" relaxation, in order to distinguish it from the more passive "static" relaxation that has come to be associated with inactivity. The balance is a dynamic, rather than static, equilibrium. This is clarified by the following example:

- Place two equal weights equal distances from the center of a seesaw and the seesaw will sit balanced if it is not disturbed. This balance is static.
- Place two chemical solutions in a beaker, one of which is producing chemical X at the same rate as the other is using chemical X, and you have a dynamic equilibrium. There is always the same amount of chemical X but it is constantly being created and destroyed. This is dynamic equilibrium.

In other words, dynamic relaxation recognizes that there are some processes in the body, mind, and emotions that tend to create a stressed condition and some that tend to create a static, relaxed condition, and that the aim is not to eliminate one set of tendencies but to bring these tendencies into balance.

Having got this far, we can now re-examine the concept of stress. Just as we found the concept of relaxation has come to mean the extreme of static relaxation, we find that the word "stress" has come to mean "excessive stress," implying that any stress is bad for the body. This is certainly not the case. All of the body's systems require a certain amount of stress in order to maintain tone and functionality. The saying "use it or lose it" is quite true.

As just one example, failure to maintain muscle tone means that the body starts to break down muscle tissue as being unwanted. Since muscle tissue is the "fourth pump" of the cardiovascular system (the other three being the heart, arterial system, and lung pump), the collapse of this system puts excessive stress on the other systems. (Inactivity also depresses the effectiveness of the lung pump, further aggravating the situation.)

To avoid the negative connotations associated with the word "stress," let us replace it with "stimulation," since there is still a clear distinction between stimulation and over-stimulation. (The word "stimulation" has neutral-to-positive associations.) We will refer to the "relaxation response" as the "calming response" and the "flight or fight response" as the "stimulating response."

Just as there must be an adequate amount of physical stimulation of the muscular system in order to maintain muscle tone, the mental and emotional capacities must be stimulated if they are not to wither and die. Dynamic relaxation therefore becomes the balance between the calming and stimulating responses.

Perhaps we could see stimulation as the yang process and calming as the yin process, with dynamic relaxation as the bringing into balance of these opposite but complementary processes. This is much more in accord with basic Chinese philosophy — seeking to balance and harmonize, rather than eliminate, processes.

Before we look at the techniques for achieving dynamic relaxation, we need to understand a little more about the human body and the way in which it functions.

DYNAMIC RELAXATION AND THE HUMAN BODY

The human body has evolved to cope with the differing requirements of long-term and short-term survival.

Short-term survival occurs when the body is under immediate threat by a predator, attacker, or natural event (a flood, fire, avalanche, etc). Here the sole focus is on surviving the next few minutes. If survival entails the body suffering some long-term damage which may lessen its longevity, so be it; all resources are thrown into the needs of the moment. This is known as the "flight or fight response." As previously mentioned (since we have little need to flee or fight these days), we will refer to this as the "stimulating response," that which shifts the body into "ready for action" mode.

Long-term survival depends on the continued functioning of the various components of the body — the musculo-skeletal system, circulatory system, internal organs, immunological systems, etc. Such functioning depends on the internal distribution of nutrients, the removal of wastes, and all systems operating within tolerance limits and not being exposed to excessive stimulation of a short-term or long-term nature. This state is known as the "relaxation" or "calming" response.

The negative impact of short-term survival responses is an acceptable trade-off when it leads to continued survival of an organism (such as lifting a car or other heavy object from an injured person) or the production of peak performances. (Athletic peak performances are a matter of debate, since the fact that athletes live no longer than average, as evidenced by life actuarial tables, indicates the health benefits from their training programs are traded off against the cost of those peak performances.)

When the stimulating response is present and there is no short-term threat or challenge, the body's systems suffer unnecessary damage, which may significantly shorten life expectancy through a system failure, or infection by external pathogens.

Unfortunately, the types of stressors experienced in the modern world are not only stressors that activate the stimulating response, they do not provide the opportunity for *release* of that response. Thus, the contemporary person may experience such responses for extended periods, with significant damage to the body's systems for no apparent trade-off benefit.

There are two physiological systems which enable the body to experience the stimulating response or the calming response:

* the autonomic nervous system; and
* the endocrine system

The autonomic nervous system

The autonomic nervous system consists of those nerves that relay the responses which are largely outside the control of the conscious mind. It is composed of two complementary systems: the sympathetic nervous system and the parasympathetic nervous system.

The sympathetic nervous system is the part of the autonomic nervous system which triggers the stimulating response. This:

* shifts blood supply away from internal organs, skin, and digestive processes to the musculoskeletal system. It does this by closing down the fine capillary networks which interlace body tissues, reducing nutrient supply, and allowing build-up of wastes and toxins in those tissues;
* raises blood pressure and increases pulse rate;
* increases oxygenation and sugar levels in the blood;
* boosts energy-producing metabolic processes, which is reflected in increased core body temperature;
* increases the rate of respiration;
* suppresses immunological responses; and
* slows down digestive processes, including the production of saliva.

11

The general result can be likened to hard acceleration when driving a car. You may go fast for a while, which is useful in avoiding collisions, but your engine suffers significant wear and tear.

The parasympathetic nervous system operates completely differently. In general terms, it reverses the above processes. It opens up the circulatory systems of the body and normalizes blood pressure, oxygenation, and sugar levels. Resistance to infection rises, and the body's healing and digestive processes work more effectively.

This all sounds marvellous, but you can have too much of a good thing. If the parasympathetic system is overly dominant, one can get what has been called the "possum response." Here, when faced with a threatening situation, the person basically does not react. There is decreased physiological functioning, loss of musculoskeletal tone, mental lassitude, inactivity, and depression. This is why the concept of dynamic relaxation, which balances these two systems and the endocrine secretions, is so important.

The sympathetic and parasympathetic nervous systems are always in operation; left to themselves they create a homeostatic balance. The trigger which raises and lowers the level of activity of these two systems appears to be the background emotional state of the mind. When we are worried, tense, angry, or fearful, the parasympathetic system activity is increased; when we are calm and happy with a feeling of well-being, the sympathetic nervous system is stimulated.

It does appear that the level of balance to which the sympathetic and parasympathetic systems return can be changed over time in response to constant stimulation and/or suppression of one of the systems. If you are generally anxious and have a nervous disposition, regularly activating the calming response can help to alleviate these symptoms.

If you live a generally unstressed life but are lethargic and unemotional, focus more on activating the stimulating response (but be careful not to confuse lethargy with fatigue from an overstressed life). Chinese health exercise systems work on rebalancing both responses.

The endocrine system

The endocrine system is a series of glands which produce various secretions that have a similar effect on the human body to that caused by activating the sympathetic and parasympathetic nervous systems. In this case, it is the production of different secretions that activate either the stimulating response or the calming response. One interesting aspect of the endocrine system is that it can act directly on the body's physical systems or indirectly through influencing mood or well-being.

For instance, the production of adrenalin directly activates the stimulating response, while production of seratonin creates a sense of well-being that triggers the calming response through the activation of the parasympathetic system. Again, the production of these secretions appears to rely on our underlying mental state. Thus, there is something of a "chicken and egg" question about where the effect starts.

Why two systems?

Why are there two systems in place to control both the calming response and the stimulating response? One could speculate that the response of the autonomic nervous system is likely to be more immediate than that of the endocrine system, as electro-chemical messages can be distributed faster through the body than can chemical secretions. On the other hand, the effects of the endocrine system are likely to be longer-lasting, as the chemical secretions produced by the endocrine system tend to remain in the system until used by the chemical processes involved in the response.

The existence of the two control systems may also be part of the way in which the body maintains its homeostatic balance, thus avoiding the triggering systems spiralling out of control.

The relaxation feedback loop

We have seen from our examination of the endocrine and autonomic nervous systems that it is our state of mind which triggers these systems into either the stimulating response or the calming response. However, the process does not stop there; there is then a feedback loop from the body to the mind. When the muscles of the body are relaxed, when the breathing is deep and gentle, the neural messages feeding back to the brain create a mental sense of well-being, which further triggers the relaxation response.

That is, there is a positive feedback loop. When we feel better emotionally, we feel better physically, which, in turn, makes us feel still better emotionally. On the other hand, when we feel tense and unhappy, our muscles tense and our breathing becomes shallower. The neural messages feeding back to the brain make us feel more tense and unhappy, further triggering the stimulating response, and so on.

It is not surprising we have mood swings, but it is surprising they do not continually spiral out of control. However, the existence of these feedback loops presents us with a number of opportunities for initiating the calming or stimulating response, either at mind or body level.

DYNAMIC RELAXATION AND THE MENTAL STATE

Our sense of well-being and our mood come from the subconscious. This can make it appear as though our mood is something outside our control. However, we have learned that our subconscious can be programmed either positively or negatively.

If we visualize positive outcomes and feelings in our conscious mind, the subconscious picks up on these messages and reflects them in our mood and sense of well-being. (This is why, if we want to benefit both mind and body, the mental imagery behind exercise movements is so important for us to know and to use.)

We have said that the calming response is not under direct conscious control, but rather that the conscious mind can influence the creation of either the calming or stimulating response by the mood it encourages the subconscious to create. It is all very well to talk about creating a mood, but how do we do it?

First, never underestimate the power of the conscious mind to involve itself directly in the workings of the body. Our pulse, blood pressure, body temperature, and rate of respiration are all responses generally handled subconsciously, yet science has found that the ordinary person can exert an amazing level of conscious control over these functions.

People have been taught, by the use of biofeedback equipment, to refine their level of control to the cellular level; a single neuron can be selected and activated. How does the mind zero in on one neuron? We have no idea. On the other hand, conscious thought can influence the simultaneous firing of millions of neurons which change the brainwave states from Beta to Alpha or Theta. While the techniques are known, the mechanisms remain mysterious.

We often accuse optimists of looking at the world through rose-colored glasses. When we do this, we forget that human beings are not machines simply recording external stimuli and performing mathematical computations on them. Human beings form a picture of the world; it has to be some color! Perhaps too many of us have a set of gray glasses. The fact is, there is no true way of looking at the world. If we consciously look for the positive in events, then our subconscious takes its cue from this, and creates a positive mood and a sense of well-being. On the other hand, if we prefer to be pessimistic and negative, our subconscious will create a mood to match.

There are many books on the power of positive thinking, on learning to be optimistic in your approach. What Chinese health exercises do is incorporate some of that basic theory into the way the exercises are performed.

Use visual imagery that evokes pleasant responses; concentrate on how you feel. The movement techniques will ensure you feel better, even if it may take a little time to feel good. The mere fact that you are paying attention to your body makes a difference. The old Chinese philosophy is that the body's chi responds both to the mood of the mind and to its conscious direction through the use of appropriate imagery; where the mind goes, the chi follows. (However, the mind does not sit back and command, it must lead by example. If you want to lead chi into your hands, then you must focus your awareness on the hands.)

RELAXATION AND PAIN

We must also consider pain. Contrary to how we sense it, pain occurs in the brain, not at the point of injury or damage. This is easily proved by stopping the signals that cause pain while they are on their way from the site of the injury to the brain, which is what occurs when we use a local anesthetic and pain is no longer felt. That pain is a mental state is particularly obvious when we suffer emotional pain; it can hurt as much, if not more, than pain from injury.

Why should nature have evolved a mental state that is so unpleasant? The answer lies in the fact that if an organism continues to injure its body unnecessarily it is not likely to survive as well as an organism that avoids pain unless it is absolutely necessary. It is nature's warning system, essential to alert the brain to activities which are injurious and to provide an incentive to avoid damaging or painful actions.

If pain is a survival mechanism, there should be override mechanisms to ensure that pain does not become contra-survival. This pain survival system is the body's natural production of its own opiates, which suppress pain and provide a mental high. (Drugs such as heroin and morphine attach themselves to the opiate receptors in the brain, imitating the natural chemicals but with horrendous side effects.)

These natural pain suppressants seem to be produced in two instances. The first is when the stimulating (flight or fight) response has run its course and the parasympathetic system is, again, in the ascendant. This is a pro-survival characteristic — the person or animal has escaped its danger and is now resting or recovering. Pain no longer has survival benefits; rather, it will interfere with the recovery process and so is suppressed.

In the second instance, survival sometimes requires prolonged action, such as running from a predator. Subjecting the escapee to extended periods of pain would seem counterproductive and we do, indeed, find there is what athletes refer to as a pain barrier. Once this is crashed through, there is a flood of natural opiates and pain is suppressed. The difference here is that damage to the body is still continuing. Over time, abuse of this survival response reduces the healthy bodies of athletes to shattered wrecks. The so-called "runner's high" is dangerous because it is psychologically addictive, with runners seeking out body-damaging conditions in order to experience the high that goes with them.

It should be appreciated that endorphins, the name given to these natural opiates, are not just physical pain suppressers. They suppress mental, emotional, and, one would suspect, spiritual pain and are mood-altering chemicals. This is fine if they are providing respite for recovery, but not if damage is still being experienced.

We may ask ourselves, why does there seem to be so much emotional and physical pain in the world today? Drug companies make fortunes selling drugs to relieve emotional pain such as depression; millions suffer the chronic pain of arthritis, back pain, or other degenerative conditions. The clue might lie in the fact that this pain is indicating there is something contra-survival in the way we are constructing our lifestyles. Survival is always about the species, not the individual. If the species in general is suffering pain, then the species as a whole has a problem. The solution therefore lies not in suppressing the pain but in identifying the root causes and eliminating them.

CONCLUSION

You now have all the theory you need to understand the concept of dynamic relaxation and its philosophy as the basis of Chinese health exercise systems. To be useful, the theory must, of course, be applied. There are two ways this can be done:

First, you could elect to apply this theory directly to such Chinese health exercise systems as:

- Shibashi Qigong;
- Tai Chi;
- Lotus Qigong;
- Tao Yin;
- Lohan Qigong;
- Yin Yang Sword; and
- Dragon Phoenix Fan.

Second, you may wish to direct your attention to some specific area of interest in, or problem involved with, your:

- posture;
- breathing;
- musculature;
- joints; or
- movement dynamics.

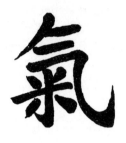

Chapter Two

Chi

CHI, OR LIFE ENERGY, is obtained from the food we eat, the water we drink, and the air we breathe; the quantity and quality of chi in these life necessities is a reflection of the overall health of our environment. The difference made by a proper supply of chi is dramatic. Symptoms of short supply, or low quality, of chi include: feeling tired and listless, sleeping poorly, low creativity and productivity, difficulty in coping with disease and infection, chronic fatigue, depression, and irritability. However, when we have an abundance of high-quality chi, life feels good, we are energetic and vital, our work is productive and creative, our relationships with others blossom, and we are much more resistant to disease and infection.

Learning to manage chi is one of the most important life skills we can acquire, yet, to date, chi has been largely ignored by modern society. However, the basic chi management skills and techniques that you need to know are quite simple; there is nothing esoteric about them and no special knowledge or abilities are required. You will probably find you are already practicing quite a number of the techniques outlined, and so you can learn to hone those skills, as well as develop chi management skills, in areas you may have overlooked.

The good news is that managing your chi properly does not require you to become a monk, or otherwise separate yourself from the normal activities of a person living in a contemporary society.

Managing your chi changes not so much *what* you do, as *how* you do it.

Because managing chi and using its power can transform your life, it is important you understand what chi is, how it functions, and how it can be controlled. It is possible simply to practice the techniques outlined, but without a basic understanding of chi, the management techniques applied might not be appropriate to the situation. We shall therefore look at the following:

- what is chi?;
- how we can see the world from a chi perspective;
- how chi works in living things;
- chi and its impact on our daily lives; and
- chi management tools.

WHAT IS CHI?

There is no English word which captures the full essence of the meaning of chi. Literal translations, such as breath, energy, and air, are fairly limited in the images and meaning they convey. Perhaps the best we can do is to speak of life energy. Chi, or life energy, is an animating force that drives not only living things but all the developmental and growth processes in the universe — from the growth of a crystal to the birth of a star or galaxy. Chi is the breath of the universe.

All this is very poetic, but what form does chi take? Is it solid, liquid, gas, or something different? The ancient Chinese often described chi as a fluid that, within the human body, flowed through a system of vessels known as *jing luo*. The *jing luo* system is (at least) as complex and detailed in structure as the blood circulatory system. The oriental health sciences of acupuncture, acupressure, and moxibustion (to name but a few) are based on various ways of stimulating the chi flows within this system.

Modern science has been unable to identify any physical vessel structures within the human body which equate to the *jing luo* system, leading to the belief that this system may be an energetic, rather than physical, structure. Modern science already knows of other energies, such as electricity and magnetic fields, that demonstrate similar qualities to those which the ancient Chinese identified as being associated with chi.

It is not hard to understand why the ancient Chinese explained chi in terms of the world with which they were familiar, and it is interesting to see how consistent the behavior of chi is with the behavior of other, more well-known, energies. For instance, magnetic fields have complex structures built of lines of force that require no physical structure, such as a vessel or wire, to support them. It is, in fact, helpful to think of chi as similar to a magnetic field, and thus imagine the universe filled with a life field that has flows of chi energy along the equivalent of lines of force.

It is worthwhile emphasizing the dual nature of chi—its existence both as a field and as a flow of energy. When we speak of chi we include both chi energy fields and chi energy flows. Most of us would probably remember our schooldays when we were given a sheet of paper with iron filings poured on it and told to place a magnet under the paper. Immediately the iron filings formed up in patterns, demonstrating the lines of force running through them from the magnetic field. The chi field is also able to organize matter that exists within its chi field.

The *jing luo*, then, should be seen not as physical structures but as energy trajectories, similar in nature to lines of force. These lines of force also exist within the general environment. The Chinese used to refer to these environmental energy pathways as dragon veins, a poetic description that brings to mind the image of chi as the dragon's blood. This imagery is used to great effect in the art of Feng Shui. There is no reason to believe that the character of the chi energy pathways in living organisms is any different from the character of the energy pathways that exist throughout nature.

The relationship of the flow of chi to the chi field is like the relationship of electricity to magnetic fields. The flow of an electric current creates a magnetic field; the rotation of a magnetic field around a conductive material, like an electric wire, creates an electric current. Electricity and magnetism are so linked that scientists talk of electromagnetism to describe the whole effect. We should think of chi in the same way — as a life field that generates flows of chi within lines of force, or dragon veins; of flows of chi which generate chi fields — the flow and the field inseparable from each other.

While Western science has not detected the existence of physical vessels corresponding with the *jing luo* system, it *has* confirmed that acupoints on the chi energy trajectories of living organisms have substantially different electro-potentials to the tissues surrounding those acupoints, and that these areas of varying electro-potential are consistent in location within and even between species.

When trying to visualize chi fields, magnetism is a useful analogy. Each atom has its own magnetic field. When the magnetic fields of atoms within an object become aligned, we have a magnet which generates a magnetic field large enough that its properties can easily be observed. Strengthen the individual atomic magnetic fields in a magnet and the overall field is strengthened.

When we breathe in air or drink water we are necessarily absorbing chi fields at the atomic level. The picture is less clear for foods and complicated chemical structures: is it only the chi fields at an atomic level or are more complicated chi fields being absorbed? The Chinese have theorized that the second possibility is, indeed, the case; and this has important implications for the way we grow and raise our food. It also has important implications for the art and environment we create around us.

The first step is to form a mental picture of what chi is; the next step is to understand the role chi plays within our lives. To do this, we really have to look at the world from a different perspective.

SEEING THE WORLD FROM A CHI PERSPECTIVE

For those who follow traditional Chinese beliefs, chi is part and parcel of their lifestyle and culture; it is how they relate to their everyday world. For example, if a child has a sore throat, the parents see it as the child's energy system overheating and would set about restoring balance to the energy system by giving the child cooling drinks, such as chrysanthemum tea. In Chinese calligraphy and painting, the beauty and worth of a work is often judged on whether it exhibits chi and spirit. The primary goal of physical exercise is to cultivate and develop the energy within. Externally, the environment is seen as filled with abundant energy, which is not only vital for our respiration but also affects our psyche. Feng Shui can be defined as the Chinese art of living and harnessing this environmental chi energy for health, happiness, and prosperity.

Despite the latest scientific discoveries, which support an energetic view of the world, the average Westerner tends to see the world from the material, Newtonian viewpoint. It is *things* that matter, with energy playing a secondary role. The announcement of the discovery of a new chemical with healing properties would be received by the public with little apprehension; the discovery of a new energy with healing properties would probably be received with concern and suspicion. Energies represent the unknown, the unreal.

How do we change this? Obviously it takes time to modify the way we see the world. The major step in learning to manage chi is to see the world as those who follow traditional Chinese beliefs do — as an energetic, rather than material, world.

The empty box example

An empty box (with four sides but no top or bottom) is shown to a group which is asked, "What does the box contain?" The first answer is, invariably, "nothing." When this does not satisfy, "air" or "space" are sometimes offered. After that, inspiration seems to dry up. The following points are then made to the group:

- We can see through the box, so obviously there is light energy.
- A hand does not freeze when placed in the box, so obviously there is heat or thermal energy.
- When a small object is placed in the box it drops downward, indicating the energy of a gravity field.
- When a compass is placed in the box it points to the north, indicating the presence of a magnetic field.
- When a radio is placed in the box it will play various selected channels; a small television would similarly pick up various stations. In fact, if the tip of a radio telescope were placed in the box it would detect radio noise from across the universe and even the background radiation that is thought to be the remnants of the big bang.
- Other instruments placed in the box would demonstrate the existence of various electrical currents and fields, mild levels of radioactivity, X-rays, and so on.

At this stage, the perceptions of the spectators change and they see themselves as swimming in a sea of energies. Matter becomes the secondary, and relatively rare, component of this energetic universe. It is not such a great leap to see the energy of chi as yet another component of this sea.

Many writers and thinkers have used the fish as an example of the above — a creature so at home in its watery environment it is unaware of it. Perhaps humans and their lack of awareness of the energetic sea in which they swim each day would make a far better example of it.

It is a good idea to spend a few moments each day contemplating the energetic environment around you. Sense the difference in the energetic feel of various locations and times — a busy shopping center or railway station compared to a quiet park or forest, the dawn of a new day compared to a sunset, winter compared to autumn.

HOW CHI WORKS IN LIVING THINGS

The Chinese have always seen chi as operating on three levels: heaven, earth, and humanity. Expressed a little differently, they see the earth as a planet having a chi field — living organisms have their own chi field and there is a universal chi field through which the planet moves.

We now know that when magnetic fields are rotated or moved past each other they can set up flows of electric current. Since the earth (and thus its chi field) is rotating and moving through space (and its chi field), it should come as no surprise that the Chinese identify a major flow of chi from the universal chi field to earth. This forms a circuit of energy which flows downwards from the universal chi field to earth's chi field and back again. The universal chi field is seen as the positive (yang) pole of this circuit and the earth as the negative (yin) pole. Living organisms in the earth's biosphere, while maintaining their own chi fields, are heavily influenced by this major cycle of energy. Since this energy flows in lines of force (rather than being equally distributed), some parts of the earth's surface are better from an energy point of view than others. This is the basis of Feng Shui.

The chi cycle

The natural processes of living organisms are built on cycles; thus, we have the carbon, food, and water cycles, etc. Chi is no exception. Living organisms obtain chi from their environment, use it to support their daily activities, and then return it to the environment. There are various activities that must be carried out within this cycle. All living organisms must:

- **Locate and obtain chi:** Chi is obtained from several sources — food, air, water, and what is known as prenatal chi. In these sources we are obtaining chi as fields, rather than flows, of energy. The flows of energy in the environment can influence the strength and health of these (as well as the body's) fields, and can therefore also be seen as a source of chi energy. The ancient Taoists had legends of adepts who learned to tap into this environmental chi much more efficiently, consequently having little need for food or water. From our viewpoint it is important to learn to locate and identify food, water, and air with high levels of beneficial chi.

- **"Digest" chi:** How we eat, drink, and breathe can be just as important as what we eat, drink, and breathe. We can lose much of the nutritional value of our food if we gulp it in a highly stressed state, or eat it in incorrect quantities and combinations. Likewise, breathing the best air in the world may not do us much good if, because of bad breathing techniques and poor posture, we are only taking in enough to survive.

- **"Internally circulate" chi:** The nutrients from food and the oxygen from air can only become part of the chemical and electrical processes taking place in our cells and organs if they are transported to the proper place within our bodies. The effectiveness and efficiency of our blood circulation system is therefore critical to our continued health and survival. Since all cells and organs in the body need chi to survive, it is also critical that the *jing luo*, or chi distribution system, be properly maintained. Poor health practices can cripple both the blood and chi circulation systems.

- **"Metabolize" chi:** Not only are foods broken down into basic nutrients in the body but complex chemicals are synthesized in various cells and organs. Chi can also be thought of as being taken into the body in a raw form and subsequently refined for various body uses. Learning how this process works, and what steps you can take to assist it, can benefit your health.

- **"Expend" chi:** Chi can be thought of in the same terms as money. While it is prudent to keep some in reserve for unexpected expenses, chi only has value when it is spent or used. It is the matching of chi income to chi expenditure that is important. We spend chi during our physical, mental, and emotional activities. Our ability to earn chi decreases with age, so excessive expenditure in early life can leave one truly poverty-stricken when old. Knowing the steps to take to avoid unnecessary chi expenditure and get the best value for what you spend is an important life skill.

- **Manage environmental influences**: Environmental influences don't just affect the chi in your food, air, and water, they affect the chi within you. Learning to eliminate negative environmental influences and accentuate the positive ones not only benefits you but creates a richer and better environment.

In this context, we should not overlook the quality of the chi that we put back into the environment. Chi is returned to the environment not so much as energy but as the impact our personal chi field has on other living things around us. Excessive yang conditions, such as anger, hate, and a desire to dominate, damage the chi fields around us. Similarly, excessive yin conditions, such as states of depression, sadness, and inadequacy, tend to draw energy from stronger chi fields. The energy we put into our emotions has either positive or negative effects on others; thus, people who simply indulge themselves with negative emotions should be regarded as the polluters of the chi environment.

When you manage chi properly, it isn't just your life that changes for the better — your family and friends will also benefit. Because you will be concerned about the quality of the chi ingested from your food, water, and air, you will naturally be concerned about the quality of your environment and act to benefit and maintain it. This is good for everybody.

THE CHI SYSTEM IN THE HUMAN BODY

To understand how the chi energy system works within the human body, it is necessary to become familiar with a number of terms:

Organ and extraordinary meridians

Each person's body has its own chi field. The basic structure of this field is the same for each person. To be consistent with the majority of literature on the subject, we will refer to the lines of force or energy trajectories within these human chi fields as meridians. The meridians in the body are divided up into two major groups:

- **Organ meridians**: These are associated with the health and functioning of specific organ systems. There are twelve organ meridians: heart; lungs; spleen; liver; kidneys; pericardium; small intestine; large intestine; stomach; gall bladder; bladder; and triple heater.

- **Extraordinary meridians**: These are associated with the balancing and distribution of chi energy throughout the body. There are eight extraordinary meridians: *du mai* (governing vessel); *ren mai* (conception vessel); *chong mai* (ocean vessel); *dai mai* (belt vessel); *yang chiao mai*; *yin chiao mai*; *yang wei mai*; and *yin wei mai*.

Chi flows along the meridians, along the organ meridians in a specific direction. It is better to visualize this flow as being like water or blood, as chi flows relatively slowly. This does not contradict its energetic nature; changes in magnetic fields can also be relatively slow.

Similarities in the operation of the blood and chi circulation systems

Just as the blood system has particular vessels which service particular organs and areas of the body but which combine to form one total system throughout which the blood fully flows, so too do the organ meridians service particular organs, with the chi itself flowing throughout the whole system.

Poor circulation of energy has much the same consequences as poor circulation of blood. Blockages and hemorrhages can occur in the chi system as well as in the blood system.

The blood circulation system has its major arteries and veins, which can be equated to the meridians; but, just as the majority of the blood circulation system lies in its microscopic capillary network, so too is most chi circulation through a network of small energy trajectories that permeate the body.

How can the flow of chi through a meridian be changed?

There are a number of ways the flow of chi in a meridian can be influenced:

- Mental concentration on the flow of chi, either by the individual or a trained chi practitioner. One focuses on moving an imaginary ball of chi along the pathway of the meridian or focuses, in sequence, on the major acupoints in the meridian. Both these techniques are chi meditation techniques.

- Brushing the hands lightly along the pathway of the meridian while focusing on energy movement in the meridian. This is called meridian brushing.

- Performing specific stretching movements and exercises. In a sense, chi can be compared to water in a pipe or channel. When the pipe or channel is straight, the water flows the fastest; when bent or curved, the flow is slower. Therefore, performing exercises that straighten the chi meridians stimulates a faster flow of energy.

- It should also be remembered that we are talking about a system of interconnected channels and that, by properly planned movements, one can shift chi from one channel to another. This exercise technique is known as *tao yin*. Most physical exercises will have chi effects, but the exercises in *tao yin* focus on stimulating energy in a particular meridian.

- Chinese muscle and joint massage will increase the flow of chi in the meridians running through the area being massaged; it is important that the person receiving the massage is comfortable both physically and mentally. Any stress or tension caused by overzealous application of the "no pain, no gain" philosophy may actually cause a reduction in the amount of chi flowing.

- Meridian chi flow may also be increased by stimulating the acupoints lying on the meridians. This stimulation may be achieved by acupuncture, acupressure, moxibustion (burning of moxa over the point), or by stimulation with laser or electrical current—or any combination thereof.

- Each meridian is associated with a particular frequency of vibration and color; thus the visualisation of color can stimulate energy flows in particular organ meridians. There are herbs that have specific effects on chi flow, as do certain sounds and scents.

The differences between organ and extraordinary meridians

Extraordinary meridians differ from organ meridians as follows. They:

- have no acupoints unique to themselves; rather, they share points on various organ meridians and can thus move energy between different meridians;
- are not related to any particular organ;
- do not flow in one particular direction. Rather, they flow from the area of highest concentration of chi to the area of lowest concentration. If there is no differential in energy levels between two points, there is no flow of energy;
- are regarded as being more responsive to mental states than are organ meridians.

Two of the extraordinary meridians contradict the above rules. The *du mai* (governing vessel) and *ren mai* (conception vessel) share the characteristics of both extraordinary and organ meridians in that:

- they are respectively associated with the brain and reproductive organs;
- they have their own acupoints;
- while the energy can flow in different ways in these meridians, one particular way is regarded as "normal";
- they are concerned with energy balancing in other meridians.

It is because their energy-balancing functions are so important that the *du mai* and *ren mai* are generally classed with the extraordinary meridians. While there has been much focus on the organ meridians in the West, the extraordinary meridians should also be seen as critical to the maintenance of health.

Subcategories of the extraordinary meridians

The extraordinary meridians divide into three important subcategories. Namely, those forming:

1. the microcosmic circulation;
2. the macrocosmic circulation; and
3. the additional extraordinary meridians.

- **The microcosmic circulation:** This is the name given to the energy circuit formed by the *du mai* and *ren mai*. These two meridians form the prime energy circuit on which the rest of the energy system depends. If the chi flow within the microcosmic circuit is not healthy, problems will develop elsewhere. The microcosmic circuit must always be the point of first attention in the meridians. An analogy is that this circuit represents the main line of a railway system; it would be asking for trouble to develop traffic on the branch lines if the main line was already handling its limit.

  As previously noted, the *du mai* and *ren mai* also serve as the organ meridians for the brain and reproductive organs, which is reflected in their names, originally translated as "governing vessel" and "conception vessel."

- **The macrocosmic circulation:** This, as the name would imply, is an extension of the microcosmic circuit. It includes six extraordinary meridians. This circuit of energy should be the next point of focus after the microcosmic circuit.

  The *yin wei mo* and *yang wei mo* are known as the great regulator channels, the former connecting with all the yin meridians — spleen, liver, lung, pericardium, kidney, and heart; the latter with all the yang meridians — stomach, gall bladder, bladder, large intestine, small intestine, and triple heater.

  The *yin chiao mo* and *yang chiao mo* are known as the great bridge channels, with their function being to balance the energy of the yin meridians with that of the yang meridians.

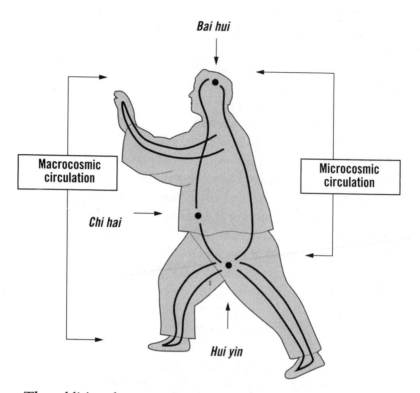

- **The additional extraordinary meridians**: These additional extraordinary meridians are of great significance. In Taoist philosophy, the *chong mai* is listed with the *du mai* and *ren mai* and they are known as the three great psychic channels. The *chong mai* (or penetrating vessel) runs from the mouth, down through/over the lungs, through the general area of the *tan tien* to *hui yin*; branches go down the legs, up through the kidneys, and along the inside of the spine. In fact, in many ways, the abdominal *tan tien* may be regarded as part of the *chong mai*, and, perhaps for this reason, the Taoists attribute to *chong mai* the capacity to store chi energy. There is considerable disputation in classical texts about the exact configuration of *chong mai*.

  The last extraordinary meridian is the *dai mai*, or belt meridian, which, apart from its general energy regulation effect, is also believed to be associated with the protection of energy in the *tan tien*.

General observations on the pathways of meridians

It must be appreciated that the meridians thread and weave their way through the human body, sometimes rising to the surface, at other times penetrating to the core. Only those portions of the meridians on the surface have accessible acupoints. Often, for the sake of simplicity and because the focus is on interacting with the existing chi flow, many books show only the accessible parts of meridian pathways. This can present a distorted view of the nature and function of the meridians.

The branches of the meridians that lie on the surface of the body are actually the least important aspect of the meridian. It is the internal part of the meridian, moving deep in the body tissue and closely associated with the internal organs, that is its vital part.

This helps clear up the confusion of how the *tan tien* connects with the meridian system. When one explores the internal pathways of the meridians, one finds that they all pass through the lower *tan tien*, which is situated just in front of the descending aorta and ascending venae cavae, immediately between the two kidneys. This area was known to the Chinese as the area of moving chi. (Since *jieng* is stored in the kidneys, the *tan tien* provides the link point between *jieng* and chi.)

Basically, when the amount of chi energy falls below the required amount, *jieng* is converted into chi, which is then available to flow through the meridian system. Whether this conversion mechanism can reverse is the subject of much speculation and disagreement. It therefore seems wise to err on the side of caution and avoid situations which tend to activate the *jieng* conversion process.

The inner trajectories of the meridians were fully specified in *The Yellow Emperor's Classic of Internal Medicine*. Modern practitioners still find these observations valid.

While, to date, there has been no conclusive identification of the bodily structures which carry chi, there is a growing belief that they are, or relate to, the fascial (connective) tissue within the body. Bio-electric currents have now been measured travelling along this tissue, and there is nothing within the structure of the fascial tissue that contradicts the energy trajectories identified by the Chinese. Since we know this tissue has connections, not only between cells but within them, it provides a communication network within the body of the same (or greater) order than the nervous system.

Acupoints

What is an acupoint?

Acupoints are specific locations on the surface of the body which have been identified as both reflecting the internal state of chi and, through various treatment methods, being able to correct and bring the body's chi into balance. Almost 1,000 such points have been identified, although knowledge of two dozen or so points is quite adequate for many basic chi management techniques.

Most of the acupoints lie on the organ meridians, but there are also some on the *du mai* and *ren mai*. Additionally, there are a small number of acupoints with no known relation to any meridian, the most well known of which would probably be *yin tang* (immediately between the eyebrows).

While the name acupoint is in common use in the West, it is misleading for a number of reasons. First, the term "acu" means needle, suggesting that the point is simply something to be needled. In actual fact, acupoints can be used for diagnosis as well as for treatment, with the sensitivity and feel of the acupoint revealing much about the underlying condition of chi. Second, there are many other applicable treatment modes (in fact, needling should be the last resort). Points can be stimulated by thought, massage, negative and positive pressure, heat and moxa, electro-stimulation and laser, and by the application of magnets. Third, the word "point" implies something minute and precisely located. Following the location description of an acupoint, however, only provides the starting point. Acupoints move within the local area and thus must be sensed or felt, not simply assumed to be in a particular location.

The original Chinese expression for acupoint was *shue*, meaning hole, cavity, or cave, which gives a much better sense of something lying hidden under the surface, which can be empty or full and which must be sought out.

Acupoint release, tonification, and sedation

The first thing to establish with any acupoint is that the chi energy can flow freely. Often, because of stress and tension within the body, the free flow of chi energy is blocked. Standard techniques are therefore intended to release or open up the point.

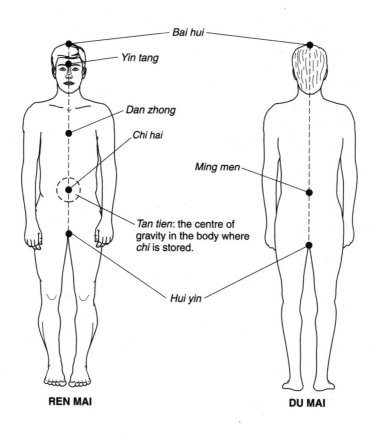

Bai hui

Yin tang

Dan zhong

Chi hai

Ming men

Tan tien: the centre of gravity in the body where *chi* is stored.

Hui yin

REN MAI

DU MAI

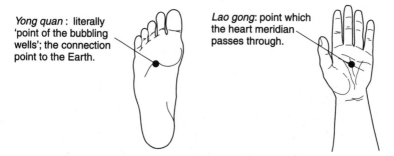

Yong quan : literally 'point of the bubbling wells'; the connection point to the Earth.

Lao gong: point which the heart meridian passes through.

Basically, opening a point is done by loosening the tissue around the point. The use of one's own chi energy can help break through a blockage. Remembering that the chi energy on organ meridians has one direction of flow, one should always work with this flow when working on any organ meridian acupoint. (No damage is done if one works opposite to the flow but neither is there any benefit.)

With the exception of the *du mai* and *ren mai*, extraordinary meridians always flow in the direction of lowest energy. These meridians have no unique acupoints and can therefore be discarded for basic acupressure work.

As mentioned, the *du mai* and *ren mai* meridians do have unique acupoints and their direction of chi energy flow can vary. In general terms, working with the direction of flow energizes and tones; working against the direction of flow calms and sedates.

Categories of acupoints

Acupoints can be divided into categories. All points in a category have similar properties.

The categories are:

- source;
- entry and exit;
- window of the sky;
- five categories;
- alarm;
- special meeting;
- four seas;
- meeting;
- tonification;
- associated;
- eight meeting;
- shokanten;
- origin and end;
- sedation;
- connecting;
- combining;
- accumulating; and
- root and side effect.

It is not intended here to explain the specific effects of these groups of acupoints, but to show that chi theory is complex. While simple techniques for toning, sedation, and treatment of everyday maladies can be used by anyone, it is a considerable leap to therapeutic application of the system, and this should only be done by a trained practitioner.

Mental stimulation of acupoints

The fact that the mind can be used to change the flow of energy at acupoints should not be surprising. Focusing attention on one point of the body often increases sensitivity (have you ever watched a mosquito bite you and distinctly felt the process of the normally undetectable bite?) and causes other physiological changes. Most people can increase blood flow and raise the temperature by at least 1°C of any point of the body on which they focus.

Tan tien

There are three *tan tien* in the human body: upper, middle, and lower. If not otherwise specified, it is the lower *tan tien* that is being referred to; it is the one with which we are most concerned while practicing breathing and Qigong exercises.

What constitutes a *tan tien* is very difficult to explain. They are not meridians or acupoints, but areas associated with particular refinements of chi energy. (Interestingly, the location of the three *tan tien* is in accordance with three of the chakras, as in yoga.)

Lower *tan tien*

This is the area which equates to the *hara*, located about three finger-widths below the navel in the center of the torso. *Tan* means pill, or immortality; *tien* means field. The *chi hai* point is at the immediate front of the *tan tien*; the *ming men* to the rear.

The *Yellow Emperor's Classic of Internal Medicine* states that the "moving chi between the kidneys" is the source of all the body's chi. What does this mean? Postnatal chi is obtained from air, food, and environment; prenatal chi is stored within the kidneys. Perhaps the expression "root of the body's chi" is more accurate.

The lower *tan tien* is seen as important because this is where the chi is stored. (However, the extraordinary meridians are also known to play the role of chi storer.) The essential role of *tan tien* may be that this is the store of energy which determines whether or not we draw on *jieng* and thus deplete our potential lifespan.

To understand the relationship between the organ meridians and the *tan tien*, imagine a set of battery-powered Christmas tree lights which are able to operate from main power when it is available but switch over to battery power when it is not. Each organ is represented by a different colored light; the wire that leads into each light is the organ meridian of that light; the transformer/battery is the *tan tien*.

Anybody who has put up Christmas tree lights knows that because the electrical circuit leads from wire to light to next wire to next light and so on, one loose connection means the whole circuit fails to work. Such a system failure would be catastrophic in a living system, and it needs something supplementary to help it overcome system faults that might develop. This is, in essence, the role of the extraordinary meridians, which act like cross-connected wires, able to take the power around faults in the system and keep the whole process going.

This explanation is, of course, simplistic. The human chi system is a lot more complicated and sophisticated, having much more in common with the national power grid and the way in which it is operated (to keep power flowing in order to meet complex sets of demands) than it does with a set of Christmas tree lights. However, the basic principle is the same.

Middle *tan tien*
In males this is located behind the sternum at the same height as the nipples; in females, a little over an inch from the base of the sternum.

Upper *tan tien*
This is located at the same height as the eyebrows, directly behind the center point between them.

Wei chi
Wei chi is another aspect of the human chi system: the strength of the human chi field to resist damage from infection and disease. If the human chi field is strong, it overwhelms the chi fields of viruses, bacteria, and other infectious agents. If the chi field is weak, these infectious agents have an opportunity to establish themselves and the human body must fall back on its other immunological defense systems.

Prenatal chi
One concept that sometimes causes a little difficulty is that of prenatal and postnatal chi. Prenatal chi is the chi inherited from the parents at the moment of conception. You will find much reference in Chinese literature to the fact that this chi is irreplaceable, that once it is gone, life ends; others argue that this energy can be replaced.

This argument can be resolved by resorting to the analogy of the national power grid, used in the discussion of the *tan tien*. If there were too great a difference between the power fed into the national grid and the power drawn out, the system would have to be shut down or it would fail physically because of damage to its component parts. Sophisticated systems are installed to prevent just such an eventuality. Even so, in countries with power shortages there are often widespread blackouts. A national power grid can be restarted, but this is rarely an option for a living system.

Prenatal chi reflects the fact that there is a minimum amount of energy necessary to keep the energy system functioning. Once we go below this, there is the risk of damage to the system, which may either shut it down permanently or impair it so that it can never again operate at its previous levels.

CHI AND ITS IMPACT ON OUR DAILY LIVES

One way or another, we are influenced by all the chi fields around us. This means that not only will our well-being be influenced by the chi consumed through our air, water, and food but by the environment in which we live. This does not mean just our physical surroundings, but the people with whom we associate and the emotions and attitudes they possess. It also means that the emotions we feel, the attitudes we take, and the manner in which we carry out our daily activities will affect the well-being of anyone with whom we come into contact.

Unfortunately, while our society has trained most of us to consider the effect of our actions on others, there has been very little (if any) training in respect to what we might term chi hygiene. We should be alert to how the quality of our chi impacts on those around us.

Keeping ourselves calm and relaxed; focusing our attention on what we are doing; making an effort to express goodwill and compassion towards others — all these improve the chi around us. Just think of the people you like to be around. What are their basic characteristics? Are they positive or negative? Do they seek to support those around them? Are they loud and aggressive, quiet and timid, or in between?

It is fascinating, indeed, that the personal qualities agreed by most people to be desirable are also those which are associated with beneficial chi. A smile, a positive thought, or a good intention are beneficial for you as well as those around you. This has always been suspected, and now we have the reason: these things affect chi.

CHI MANAGEMENT TOOLS

In order to manage chi we need to be able to describe the condition which it is actually in as well as the condition in which we would like it to be. The Chinese have had some 4,000 years to contemplate this problem, and they have come up with a very useful descriptive model known as the "five elements and ten stems" model. To understand this model, two theories must be understood:

• the yin/yang theory; and
• the five elements theory.

When we are able to identify the yin/yang condition of chi and at which stage of the five elemental energies cycle the chi is, we can draw on a wealth of observational knowledge, built up by the Chinese over millennia, which allows us to manage our chi properly.

The yin/yang theory and chi management

The yin/yang theory

Like hot and cold, yin and yang are easy to understand but difficult to explain. The best solution is simply to list those things that present as either yin or yang. Only pairs of descriptive opposite verbs can be rendered as yin/yang couplets. Any terms which involve judgment, such as "good/evil," "right/wrong," etc., would not be appropriate.

Applying the yin/yang concept to chi

Just as an electric current is said to be positive or negative, the state of chi is said to be either yin or yang. It must be remembered that yin and yang are, like cold and hot, relative rather than absolute terms; that is, something may be hot in relation to something that is colder but, at the same time, be cold in relation to something that is hotter. A hot day at the North Pole would be a cold day at the equator. Thus, you cannot call chi either yin or yang until you have compared it with something.

If identification of attributes indicates a yin/yang imbalance, there are a number of ways to correct this. Let us say, for instance, there is a mild excess of yang. Balance can be achieved by either increasing the amount of yin or reducing the amount of yang; where there is a mild deficiency of yang, the opposite approach would be taken. Where there is an extreme excess or deficiency of either yang or yin, focus would be on removing the excess or deficiency rather than seeking to balance it. Thus, not only the balance but also the relative amounts of yin chi and yang chi have to be taken into account.

The five elements theory and chi management

The translation of the name of this theory is rather misleading and has only been used because it is the name you will come across in other literature on the subject. A far better description is the five elemental phases of the energy cycle. This conveys that we are not talking about things but about stages through which energy goes. Moreover, these stages are a cycle, in that they have no beginning or end; one stage leads to the next until we come full circle.

As well as having a yin/yang condition, chi will be in one of the five phases of the energy cycle. This may sound confusing, but think of earth — it both rotates on its own axis and revolves around the sun. If you think of the yin/yang condition of chi as its rotation, passing through day and night, and the five element phases of chi as its revolution around the sun, passing through five seasons (breaking summer into two seasons, summer and high summer), then you have an analogy that may make the relationship between the yin/yang theory and the five elements theory a little easier to understand.

It should be understood clearly that the elements are only symbols of the processes that take place in each phase. Each phase can be in either a yin or yang condition.

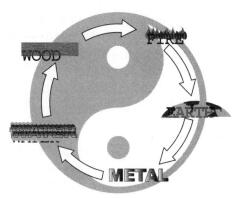

Because these energy phases underlie the functioning of the natural world, we would expect to identify many correspondences in nature with the underlying energy phase. The Chinese have, in fact, identified many such correspondences, with the major ones listed in the following table.

CORRESPONDENCE	WOOD	FIRE	EARTH	METAL	WATER
SEASON	spring	summer	high summer	autumn	winter
COLOR	green	red	yellow	white	blue
TASTE	sour	bitter	sweet	spicy	salty
SMELL	rancid	scorched	fragrant	rotten	putrid
SOUND	shouting	laughing	singing	weeping	groaning
EMOTION	anger	joy	compassion	grief	fear
DISPLAYS IN	nails	face color	lips	skin, body hair	head hair
CLIMATE	wind	heat	dampness	dryness	cold
SENSE ORGAN	eyes	tongue	lips	nose	ears
YIN ORGAN	liver	heart	spleen	lungs	kidney
YANG ORGAN	gall bladder	small intestine	stomach	large intestine	bladder

As with yin/yang attributes, it is important not to confuse the correspondences with the actual energy phase — they are simply useful tools to determine the energy phase as a basis for predicting the results of actions that we might take.

GENERAL CHI LIFE SKILLS

Chi and sleep

We tend not to think too much about sleep, unless we don't get enough of it! Scientific studies have shown, however, that there is a strong link between the quality of sleep and life expectancy. Chinese sayings in traditional medicine also indicate the early recognition of the importance of sleep:
- Sleeping and eating are the keys to preserving health.
- Those who sleep and eat well can live long.

The fact that sleep occupies roughly one third of our total lives would indicate that it plays a vital role in our health.

However, sleep seems to have a number of disadvantages in the survival game. While asleep, we cannot defend ourselves and so are vulnerable to attack. During the sleeping period, the body is using energy to sustain its metabolism but cannot undertake any food-gathering activities. It would seem that the ability to sleep for shorter periods would confer an evolutionary advantage and that nature would select for this trait. The fact that it hasn't implies greater evolutionary advantage is conferred on the organism that gets a significant period of sleep.

We know that when we get a good night's rest we waken feeling refreshed and recharged, and our sense of well-being is high. A long sleep is not necessarily required as extended periods of sleep sometimes leave us feeling sluggish and lethargic. This implies that sleep is a period of time in which the chi rebuilds but that if the sleep period is too long the chi begins to stagnate.

On the other hand, we all recognize that in cases where we attempt to sleep when physically, mentally, or emotionally exhausted (if we are successful in getting to sleep at all), we still awaken tired and with low energy levels. It would seem that sleep itself is an activity that requires a reasonable level of chi, in order to be carried out.

We have some understanding of the reason for this when we look at sleeping behavior during periods of sickness or recuperation. The body seems to increase its level of sleep automatically, and it is acknowledged that at such times this sleep helps the healing process. This is more than simply the advantage conferred by physical inactivity; lying still but awake is not nearly so useful.

Obviously, chi does not simply rebuild during sleep but participates in important rebuilding and recuperative activities. This makes sense, because sleep is a time when the chi field is most undisturbed. The ability of this field to influence the processes that are taking place in the body should therefore be at its height. This is confirmed by the fact that if we attempt to sleep in an emotionally, mentally, or physically stimulated state then, even if sleep comes, it tends to be fitful and unsatisfying.

Good sleep, then, contributes to our life expectancy, helps us resist and fight off infection, and contributes significantly to our state of well-being during the day. Obviously, it is important to ensure that our sleeping techniques help us to secure all the advantages that a good night's sleep can bring.

Chi sleeping techniques

How much sleep?

The sleep requirement for each individual is different and changes with age, as well as with activities undertaken. The best measure is how you feel when you wake up. If you are sleeping long periods of time (in excess of eight hours) but still feeling lethargic, try reducing the period of time you spend asleep. If this does not improve matters, start looking at things which are affecting your quality of sleep.

In general terms, sleep should be considered a yin activity, a period of restoration and consolidation, a gathering of energies for the next day. Accordingly, in the yang period of the year (spring and summer) there is less need for sleep, while in the yin period (autumn and winter), sleep periods may be increased. In this way, seasonal energies are synchronized with sleep requirements. Also, yang personalities generally need less sleep than yin personalities.

The important thing is that sleep periods be regular. Varying the sleep period throws out the whole cycle of energy for the day and over a period of time will be deleterious to health.

Here are some general sleep-time indicators: babies, fourteen to eighteen hours; children seven to fifteen years, ten hours; adults, eight hours; and adults eighty-years plus, nine to ten hours.

Quality of sleep

Quality of sleep depends on the condition in which you prepare for sleep, together with your sleep environment.

- **Preparation for sleep:** As previously noted, the best condition for sleep is when the chi is tranquil but not depleted. Try to avoid situations that lead to being mentally, emotionally, or physically overstimulated. (This does not include sex, since the body has its own mechanisms for inducing a relaxed state following this activity.) It is important that the body be free of stress and tension when you sleep. Performance of relaxation exercises and such activities as Tai Chi can, when performed correctly, help assist the body to prepare for sleep, particularly if there has been little physical activity during the day or considerable mental or emotional activity. Overeating prior to sleeping can lead to disturbed sleep, as can excessive consumption of alcohol. A small amount of alcohol can assist relaxation but it is best to avoid drug-induced sleep. (This includes sleeping pills, since the sleep that results is rarely beneficial.)

- **The sleeping environment**: Here we need to consider both the sleeping equipment and the sleeping room. Sleeping equipment consists of the bed, pillow, coverings, and sleeping clothes. The firmness of the bed should be selected with a view to ensuring maximum chi flow. This means that the bed should not be so firm that the weight is taken by only a few portions of the body, with consequent pressure and the reduction in the flow of chi, nor should the bed be so soft that the middle portion of the body collapses, as again, this will inhibit the flow of blood and chi. The pillow should be selected according to similar considerations. It should support the head, taking pressure off the neck, and should be firm but not too high. The pillow actually offers an opportunity for further health measures; the Chinese often fill pillows with aromatic and curative materials. Bed coverings and sleeping clothes are there to maintain a microclimate around the body, protecting it from sudden changes in temperature. It is important that the body be protected against drafts and temperature changes, as the chi is particularly vulnerable at this time. The sleeping room should be the first-line defence against excessive cold, wind, or dampness. The room should also reduce noise levels and other disturbances that would wake the sleeper. It is most important that proper ventilation be maintained, and that the air chi be of good quantity and quality. (Beware of flowers in a room at night, as they consume, rather than produce, oxygen at this time.)

Chi and relationships

By relationships, we include those with family, workmates, friends, and acquaintances. Each day we either deepen and strengthen our relationships or weaken and eventually destroy them. Since these relationships often constitute our most valued possessions, we should look closely at how the state of our chi influences others, and vice versa.

When two human chi fields come into contact, they act on each other as any other fields do. The result is that the two fields will be more similar after contact than before it. This means that when a positive chi field (from a person with a sense of well-being) meets a negative chi field (from a person who is depressed or angry), the positive field will become a little more negative and the negative field a little more positive. Where the two fields are either both negative or both positive, the fields reinforce each other and become either more positive or more negative, as the case may be.

Maintaining positive chi fields

At first glance, it might seem that the best way of maintaining your positive chi is to avoid all those with negative chi fields and this is, indeed, a solution. However, we all have days when we are depressed, and it would be unpleasant to think that on those days all happy people would avoid us so that all we had were negative people with whom to associate! On those days we need our contact with positive chi people and, in return, we need to be available for those people when they are depressed.

What we have to do is monitor the state of our well-being. When we are feeling down we should seek out positive people and avoid negative ones, otherwise we will reinforce our own problems. When we feel good, however, and we contact a negative person, we should seek to help that person attain a more positive state. This is not always possible and we should certainly be wary of associating with many negative people for extended periods.

The other point about monitoring our personal chi states is that it gives us the opportunity to do something about them. If we are depressed, we can read or watch material that will lift our spirits. (This may not be what we want to do, and so some mental effort may be involved here!) We should also try activities we know will lift our spirits.

Since our chi fields are influenced by those around us, we should be aware that, if through anger or ego, we damage one of those chi fields, we have, in effect, damaged our own chi field, however satisfactory the anger or victory may feel at the time. (In fact, very strong emotions damage the energetic system and body anyway. The Chinese say that excess joy hurts the heart, anger hurts the liver, worry hurts the spleen, sadness hurts the lungs, and fear hurts the kidneys.)

There are two other things we can do to help ensure our personal chi fields remain as positive as possible — make laughter and smiling part of our everyday lives. As one Chinese saying goes, "A laugh makes you ten years younger and worry turns your hair gray." X-ray photography of smiling people shows that the smile is accompanied by wide-ranging physiological changes, including relaxation of internal organs that may previously have been held tensely.

So, if you want your relationships to prosper: seek to maintain a relaxed and optimistic outlook by avoiding stress and worry (or taking action to reduce the effects of these); don't suppress anger but try to channel and control it, and try to avoid directing it at people (it won't achieve anything positive anyway); become aware of the well-being of the people with whom you are dealing and try to say and do things to improve it; and if you are the target of anger, hate, or any other negative emotion, try to deflect it rather than react to it.

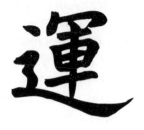

Chapter Three

Chi Breathing

HISTORY AND PHILOSOPHY

THERE IS SUCH A CLOSE CONNECTION between chi and breathing that they are sometimes described as synonymous. Food we can survive without for weeks, and water and sleep for days, but a few minutes' deprivation of breath will also deprive us of life.

Expiration is a synonym for death, inhalation for growth and development. The body seems to recognize the presence of beneficial chi automatically, and when we are in its presence we breathe deeply or slowly. Think of the times you are moved to breathe deeply: standing on a cliff, looking out at the majesty of the ocean; on a mountain top, with a beautiful panorama spread out before you. This deep breathing is not a response to oxygen levels, which are actually at their lowest at high altitude.

The atmosphere separates the earth from the rest of the universe. All energies flowing into and out of the earth must pass through it, charging it with chi energy. Furthermore, the atmosphere is the home of life and must be affected by all the living chi fields within it. (The atmosphere had to form before oceans could develop, or they would have boiled away, most of the respiration products of life in the ocean being released into the atmosphere. The plant life in the ocean is the main source of the planet's oxygen.)

The way in which we breathe affects both the quantity and quality of the chi taken into our lungs and the amount we are able to absorb into our bodies. The degree to which the lungs expand and contract is only important to chi breathing in terms of the quantity of chi to which the body has access. It is in the process of inhalation and exhalation that the chi in the air is absorbed into the body's energetic system. The parts of the energetic system most involved are the *du mai* and *ren mai* meridians, together with the *tan tien* — in other words, the microcosmic circulation.

Good chi breathing therefore means that we should be doing some things additional to, but consistent with, good physiological breathing.

APPROACH TO LEARNING
Important warning about breathing exercises
A word of warning before we look at some chi breathing techniques. Chi breathing is mainly about the mental focus we have when breathing, together with some physiological aspects such as breathing through the nose and using diaphragmatic breathing. It does not require forcing the breath or mentally overriding the depth and frequency of your breathing. Doing this can cause discomfort and can even be dangerous. Develop the art of listening (with your ears and your body) to your breath. Your breathing will change naturally as you become aware of what you are doing; there is no need to try to control it.

Taking too much air into the lungs rapidly floods the body with oxygen. This is called hyperventilation and has all sorts of negative effects. The other extreme, breathing too shallowly or too infrequently, is called hypoventilation, and can deprive the brain of the required oxygen, resulting in fainting. If you have any breathing condition, such as asthma, learning to chi breathe should help, but seek your doctor's advice first.

TECHNIQUES
Breathing through the nose
We should breathe in through the nose. From a physiological viewpoint, this filters out airborne bacteria and helps ensure air reaches lungs at a temperature and humidity most beneficial to them.

However, when we exert ourselves strenuously we breathe in through the mouth. The reason for this is simple. When our metabolism is operating at a high level, the amount of oxygen required to fuel the process goes up and we require a bigger air intake; thus we switch over to the mouth. In our evolution, this situation would have arisen when we were either obtaining food or seeking to avoid becoming food. At such times, survival is what is important and it makes sense to trade off some long-term health benefits to get through the next few moments. Besides, if we are only mouth breathing for short periods of time, the negative health aspects are not liable to be significant. The important thing to remember is that nose breathing should be used for over 95 percent of breathing.

When you go to smell something, it is as though you focus the inward breath on the inner tip of the nose. This would have been an important survival characteristic in the past, when the scent of danger or food was something we needed to know about as soon as possible, but today we rarely use this skill. This is a pity, because there is an acupoint at the tip of the nose called *su liao*, which becomes activated when we draw in air to the tip of the nose. This is the first point at which a linkage between the body's energetic systems and the air chi becomes established. When you consider the important relationship between certain aromas and our body's overall state (such as lavender providing the stimulus for relaxation), the implications of the disuse of this acupoint is something which warrants more study than it has received. There are a number of Chinese exercises (such as "Buddha Smelling Roses") which require focusing the breath on this point. Alternatively, you can incorporate the focus of air on the inner tip of the nose as part of your standard breathing visualization. The more you practice, the more likely you are to begin breathing correctly. Do not snort or sniff; the air should be taken into the nose smoothly and quietly. The key is the mental focus at the tip of the nose.

Breathing through the nose has the additional benefit of enabling the tip of the tongue to stay against the roof of the mouth. This forms a physical connection between the end of the *du mai* and the starting point of the *ren mai* meridians, thus completing the microcosmic orbit and greatly encouraging the flow of energy therein.

Chi hai

The *chi hai* acupoint (the name means "sea of chi") is perhaps the most important point involved in breathing. While the *chi hai* point lies on the *du mai*, it is the connection point for the *tan tien*, and mentally focusing on this point greatly increases the chi absorbed from breathing.

The *chi hai* lies three finger-widths below the navel. Even though air finishes its journey in the lungs, it is helpful to imagine the breath flowing downwards to this point. The visualized stream of air should mentally be followed from the nose, down the throat and then just under the skin, along the centerline of the body, to the *chi hai* point. In other words, from the base of the throat, the image of the path along which the air is flowing is the same as the trajectory of the *ren mai* — the direction of both breath and chi flow is the same.

Diaphragmatic breathing
Diaphragmatic breathing has, as well as all its useful physiological benefits, a stimulatory effect on the *tan tien*. The inward movement of the abdomen with the outbreath and the outward movement with the inbreath are good indications of the proper movement of the lung diaphragm.

Unfortunately, the lung diaphragm is particularly susceptible to stress and tension and it may take some time to relax this area and get the diaphragm to do its job. The benefits are worthwhile and include (apart from chi advantages):
- greatly increased lung capacity;
- internal massaging effects on the internal organs, which improve their blood circulation, resulting in their obtaining more nutrients and getting rid of waste products more efficiently. This improves the health and functioning of the internal organs, which is vital to overall health;
- internal massaging effects on the large and small intestine, which assist the peristaltic process and improve the efficiency of digestion; and
- internal massaging effects on the lymphatic system. This is a key part of our immunological defence system and its circulation relies on these internal massaging effects, provided primarily by lungs and muscles.

When the lung diaphragm is functioning fully (and not before), one can involve the pelvic diaphragm. This should be raised on each inbreath and lowered on each outbreath — the reverse of the lung diaphragm.

Because this increases compression in the area between the two diaphragms, there should be an increased outward movement of the abdominal wall.

When both diaphragms are fully functional, one can tighten the abdominal muscles on inbreath and relax them on outbreath. This maximizes the compression and internal massaging.

Any attempt to move too fast in developing this breathing will be counterproductive. Each stage must be mastered before the next is attempted.

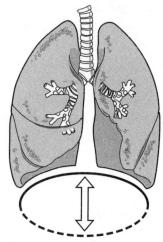

**Inbreath
Diaphragm down
Outbreath
Diaphragm up**

**DIAPHRAGMATIC BREATHING
STAGE ONE**

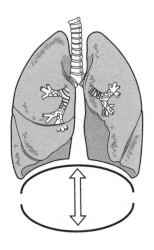

Outbreath

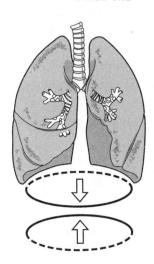

Inbreath

**DIAPHRAGMATIC BREATHING
STAGE TWO**

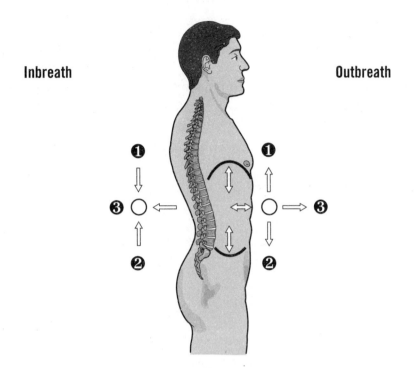

Inbreath   Outbreath

DIAPHRAGMATIC BREATHING
STAGE THREE

Exhalation

With exhalation, the air is returned from the lungs to the nose. When visualizing the flow of air, imagine the air moving up the center of the back, just under the skin, to the base of the neck. Then follow the sensation of the air, up the throat and out of the nose. In other words, the upward, outward path of the air follows the direction of the *du mai*.

A more advanced version of this breathing can be performed by initially directing the outward breath of air downwards to the *hui yin* acupoint on the perineum, then upwards along the spine to the crown of the head at the *bai hui* point and downwards again to the *su liao* point. Effectively, this breathing opens up the entire microcosmic circulation, but it is a very powerful breathing technique that may have some side effects if not approached in a controlled manner. Certainly, if you are attempting this breathing pattern and you feel any physical or mental discomfort, focus your mind on the *tan tien* and center your energy there.

Golden cloud breathing

Close your eyes and imagine yourself in the center of a glowing golden cloud. As you breathe in, imagine yourself taking in wisps of this cloud; feel the cloud warming you internally, giving you a feeling of health and vitality; feel energized. The breathing pattern is the same as your current stage of diaphragmatic breathing.

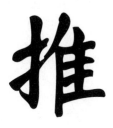

Chapter Four

Chi Massage

THE FOLLOWING CHI MASSAGE EXERCISES should be performed prior to chi meditation. (The better the mind and body feel when you perform chi meditation, the better the results.) However, they can also be used as a stand-alone exercise if you are tired or jaded. The purpose of these massage exercises is to stimulate the flow of chi, with the added benefits of improved blood circulation to the skin and enhanced skin tone.

Personal preparation
Remove glasses and any rings, watches, or jewelry that could cut or scratch. Do not perform the exercises if you have any cuts or abrasions, or have had recent surgery in the relevant area. Be cautious if you have long fingernails.

Massage set preparation
Stand in the Quiet Standing position: see pages 60–62. Relax and allow your breathing to become deep.

EXERCISES

Hand massage
Keeping the shoulders relaxed:
*   Rub the palms together in a circular motion, extending the motion until the palm and fingers of one hand pass over the palm and fingers of the other hand.

- Once the palms and undersides of the fingers are warm and gently flushed, change the movement so that the hands rub against each other from the base of the palm to the fingertips. Allow the fingers to spread so that they interweave.
- Next, interweave the tiger's mouths (the area between the thumb and index finger) and gently squeeze and loosen up the tiger's mouth areas and the sides of the fingers.
- Finally, use the palm of one hand to massage the back of the other hand, while the thumb massages the palm area. Repeat, with the hands playing opposite roles.

Dry face washing

- Place the pads of the first three fingers of each hand next to the edge of each side of the mouth.
- Push the hands gently upwards, along the sides of the nose and up to the top of the temple, then draw them downwards, along the outside of the eyes, to the jawbone and then up to the starting point.

Going up the face, the fingerpads are pushed upwards; going across the face, the fingerpads are drawn sideways; coming down, the fingerpads are drawn downwards. Keep as much of the hands in contact with the face as possible. As you draw the fingerpads downwards, press the side of the thumbs firmly in along the underside of the jaw line. The movement should be slow and even.

- If synchronizing breathing, breathe in on the upward movement and out on the downward movement.
- Repeat eight times.

Rubbing the neck

- Place the fingerpads below the jaw bone and push them backwards across the neck so that they meet behind the neck. Then draw the hands back until the fingerpads return to their starting position.
- Breathe in as you push hands backwards, breath out as you draw hands back.
- Repeat eight times.

Brushing the arms

- With the arms hanging loosely by your sides, shake them gently so that the whole arm vibrates.
- Extend the left arm forwards, at about heart height, with the palm facing downwards and the shoulder relaxed. Place the tiger's mouth of the right hand at the top of the left arm, just below the shoulder, and, squeezing gently with the thumb and fingers, brush the hand down along the length of the arm to the fingertips.
- Repeat eight times.
- Turn the palm to face upwards and repeat, this time brushing the underside of the arm.
- Repeat eight times.
- Repeat the whole sequence on right arm.
- Breathe in as you prepare, breathe out as you brush downwards.

Brushing the legs

- Transfer body weight onto the left leg, then gently shake the right foot and leg so that the whole leg vibrates. Change legs and repeat.

The remainder of the exercise can be done from either a sitting or standing position, or by placing one foot on a bench or chair.

- Place the hands on either side of the left leg. The thumbs are together, the fingers curled around the leg with fingertips pointing towards each other. Squeezing gently, push the hands down the leg and along the foot and toes.
- Repeat eight times.
- Then repeat on right leg.
- Breathe in as your prepare, breathe out as you brush downwards.

Moving chi in the abdomen

- Interlock the fingers and place them just under the left ribs.
- Pressing the hands firmly into the abdomen, draw them across the abdomen to just under the right ribs.
- Pressing inwards with the heels of the hands, push them downwards to the right pelvic bone.

- Now draw the hands firmly across the body to the left pelvic bone, pressing inwards.
- Release the pressure and glide the hands upwards to the starting position.
- Repeat eight times.
- Breathe in as you bring the hands upward and across. Breathe out as you bring the hands downward and across.
- Tighten the buttocks as you breathe in. Release as you breathe out.

Quiet standing with golden cloud visualization

- Bring the interlocked fingers over the *tan tien* area.
- Imagine yourself surrounded by a glowing, golden cloud.
- As you breathe in, take wisps of this cloud into your lungs. It feels warm and exhilarating but at the same time peaceful and relaxing.
- With each inbreath you feel better, until you are feeling totally healthy and relaxed.

You can finish the exercise sequence here or move into the chi meditation.

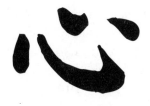

Chapter Five

Chi Meditation

HISTORY AND PHILOSOPHY

THE MIND HAS THE ABILITY TO MOVE the chi around the body. This should not really be surprising; even such an august publication as the *Scientific American* has reported experiments where the simple act of focusing the mind on a beaker of water has succeeded in creating a measurable rise in the temperature of that water.

We can therefore use mind-focusing techniques to improve the circulation of chi within the body. Additional benefits derived from this type of focusing include those that flow from any form of directed meditation; that is, improved concentration and reduction of stress.

Meditation is a word that is often misunderstood. Basically, it means to keep your mind focused on one activity; feelings of being calm and centered are by-products of it. If your thoughts are truly centered on one activity, you cannot also be worrying about the success or failure of the activity, or the time allowed for it, or any other distracting thought. So, when the mind reaches one point of focus, other worries naturally drop away and you become mentally and physically calm.

Some people believe that meditation is thinking about nothing, but this is actually a contradiction in terms. If you were told not to think about a green horse, the only way you could be sure of doing this would be to hold in your mind the thought that you were not thinking about a green horse. Replace the words "green horse" with nothing and the contradiction becomes more apparent.

Many people go to sleep when they try to practice allowing their minds to drift; they are focusing on turning off the conscious mind and they succeed. Others, who remain awake, become frustrated that their conscious minds exhibit consciousness by retaining a state of awareness, with distracting thoughts continually drifting across them. Such "meditation" is not likely to be relaxing and, in fact, can be quite stressful.

The history of meditation is probably as old as the conscious human mind. The Chinese, as usual, developed their own approach. First, they focused on the fact that the mind had what we refer to in the West as "right" and "left" brain aspects. In Chinese terms these were the yang *"yi,"* the part of the brain that dealt with logical, rational thought and that housed intellect, memory, and willpower, and the yin *"shen,"* which dealt with emotion and feeling and was the source of intuition and creativity. Meditation was about developing and harmonizing all these aspects through directed activity.

Given that the Chinese see these brain aspects as energy states based on the body's refined chi, it is understandable that they would regard the development, refinement, and transportation of chi as important aspects of meditation. Together the techniques used to achieve these processes became known as chi meditation.

The Chinese also thought more in terms of a body-mind entity than of a separate mind and body. For instance, the emotional aspects of *shen* were based on the energetic condition of various organ systems. Therefore, whereas the meditation systems of many other cultures viewed the body as a distracting nuisance that had to be ignored or dominated, the Chinese saw the body as an integral part of the meditative process. Thus, chi meditation techniques are actually body-mind meditative techniques that pay attention to all aspects of the body, be they physical, energetic, intellectual, or emotional.

Chi meditation is based on a particular theory of chi generation, energetic circulation, storage, and transformation (although it can be practiced quite successfully without detailed knowledge of these).

PRINCIPLES

The principles of chi meditation are:
- environment;
- postures;

- breathing; and
- visualization.

Environment

The area in which you perform your meditation should be free from drafts and extremes of temperature. It should have a fresh flow of air and be as quiet as possible. (Exterior disruptive sounds can be masked by music or the sound of water, such as from an indoor fountain.) Naturally, the better the environmental chi, the better the effects of the meditation.

A *si jian* Feng Shui examination can be performed to determine the environmental chi condition: see discussion of Feng Shui in Chapter 7.

Clothing should be considered to be part of the environment. Basically, make sure it is loose and comfortable, and protects you from drafts or changes in temperature.

Chi meditation postures

There are innumerable postures that can be used for chi meditation but they basically belong to three types:

- quiet standing postures;
- sitting postures; and
- energy enhancing postures.

Each posture has its own particular advantages and these are detailed in Techniques. You will note that no reference has been made to lying postures. The reason for this is as follows. The major chi circulation system in the body consists of the *du mai* and *ren mai* meridians. The circulation of chi in this system is maximized when the spine is vertical and extended, with the head lifted as though through the crown of the skull and the coccyx tucked under. This is very difficult to achieve in a lying position. Further, especially when lying on your back, the internal organs are incorrectly positioned — the contents of the abdominal cavity press back against the diaphragm and inhibit proper breathing. The greater chi circulation system is, if anything, even harder to activate properly while lying downwards.

Kneeling and lotus-type postures, where you sit cross-legged, also tend to cut the circulation of energy, especially when you are unfamiliar with these positions.

Breathing

Breathing is a most important aspect of chi meditation — it helps to focus and direct the chi. There are a number of techniques that can be used but the best initially is diaphragmatic breathing: see Chapter 3.

Visualization

The use of the mind to direct the chi, by focusing on acupoints and meridians, stimulates the flow of chi in those areas.

APPROACH TO LEARNING

Many Chinese exercise programs incorporate the basic elements of chi meditation, and a grounding in them would be given as part of the teaching of the Shibashi, Tai Chi, Lotus, mind-power Qigong, and Lohan techniques.

APPROACH TO PRACTICE

Time requirements for chi meditation

The first thing you need to do is set aside a time and place for practice. One continuous period of fifteen to twenty minutes of chi meditation per day can be most beneficial. Chi meditation can be carried out at any time during the day, but early mornings are especially good — it is the yang phase of the day and your body energy is beginning to mobilize.

Do not perform chi meditation immediately after a heavy meal, when you are hungry or physically or mentally exhausted, or when you are deeply depressed, angry, or upset. In these instances, the Quiet Standing exercise is much better: see below.

Clothing for chi meditation

Clothing should be loose and comfortable, and sufficient to prevent the body becoming chilled. Remove anything which impedes the free flow of chi within the body, such as rings and watches. Do not forget the feet; loose slippers or Kung Fu shoes allow proper circulation of chi and blood.

TECHNIQUES

Quiet Standing

Also known as Standing Zen.
First, establish the physical posture.

- The feet are parallel and shoulder-width apart, the toes pointing to the front.
- The weight of the body is equally distributed over each foot and centered in the sole of the foot; that is, do not rock forward onto the toes or carry more than 50 percent of the weight on the heels. Allow the whole foot to relax as much as possible.
- The knees are bent to a comfortable degree and point in the same direction as the toes.
- If you lower yourself too far, muscle tension will distract you from your meditation.
- The pelvic area is open. Visualize the pelvis as a large bowl and try to keep it horizontal. This can often be achieved by tilting the coccyx forward (which also reduces the strain on the lumbar area of the back).
- Now visualize yourself as suspended from the center of the crown of the head. The jaw is relaxed, tucked slightly downwards, and inwards.
- The shoulders are relaxed and the arms hang loose at the sides. To open up the shoulder joint, turn the palms to face the rear. The fingertips are gently extended, with the tiger's mouth (the area between the thumb and index finger) open. Make sure the shoulders are at equal height and face forward, preventing bowing or twisting of the spine.
- The chest and abdomen are relaxed and the spine is straight.
- The eyes are relaxed and looking straight ahead. Rather than looking at something, let whatever is in front of you come into your line of vision. This will prevent you from focusing too strongly.
- The lips are lightly together but the teeth are separated, with the tip of the tongue resting on the upper palate.

Now move on to the mental posture:
- Relax and focus on the *tan tien*. Imagine yourself breathing down to this area and out to the tip of the nose. Make sure your abdomen is relaxed — feel it moving outwards with each inbreath, inwards with each outbreath.

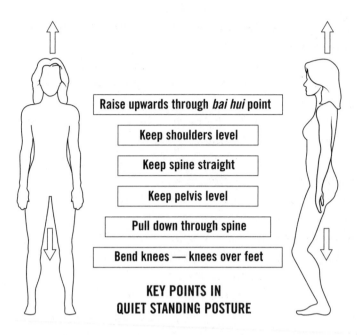

Raise upwards through *bai hui* point

Keep shoulders level

Keep spine straight

Keep pelvis level

Pull down through spine

Bend knees — knees over feet

**KEY POINTS IN
QUIET STANDING POSTURE**

- After you have established your breathing pattern, focus on your body and observe what happens — to your shoulders, your chest, your spine, your throat, and your scapulae — each time you breathe.

Quiet Sitting

Take a stool or chair. (If using a chair, use one in which the seat is firm and does not slope backwards.) The height should be such that when you sit with the base of the spine close to the front edge of the chair, the feet rest comfortably on the floor, with the upper part of the leg horizontal and the lower part of the leg vertical.

- Sit without touching the back of the chair or stool. The spine should be kept upright.
- The feet should be placed flat on the ground about shoulder-width apart, feet parallel and toes pointing to the front. The upper part of the legs should be horizontal and the lower legs perpendicular, so that the small amount of weight resting on the legs is distributed equally on both feet and over the heel and base of the toes.
- The head should be as though lifted by a string from the

center of the top of the head (the *bai hui* acupoint). The jaw is relaxed and tucked slightly inwards and downwards.

- The shoulders and elbows should be relaxed, palms resting on the upper thighs. The fingertips are gently extended and the tiger's mouth (the area between the thumb and index finger) is open. Make sure the shoulders are at equal height and face forward, preventing bowing or twisting of the spine.
- The chest and abdomen are relaxed and the spine is straight.
- The eyes are relaxed and looking straight ahead. Rather than looking at something, let whatever is in front of you come into your line of vision. This will prevent you from focusing too strongly.
- The lips are lightly together but the teeth are separated, with the tip of the tongue resting on the upper palate.

Now move on to the mental posture:

- Relax and focus on the *chi hai* point. Imagine yourself breathing down to it and out to the tip of the nose. Make sure your abdomen is relaxed and feel it moving outwards with each inbreath, inwards with each outbreath.

**KEY POINTS IN
QUIET SITTING POSTURE**

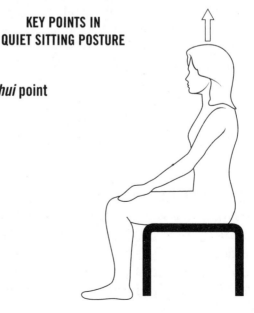

**Raise upwards through *bai hui* point
Keep shoulders level
Keep spine straight
Keep pelvis level
Knees over feet
Feet shoulder-width apart**

- After you have established your breathing pattern, focus
  on your body and observe what happens — to your
  shoulders, your chest, your spine, your throat, and your
  scapulae — each time you breathe.

ENERGY ENHANCING

There are many options for enhancing energy, the simplest of which
would be to perform the meditation in the horse-riding stance (that is,
standing with the knees slightly bent, as though you are in the saddle).
However, you must be comfortable in this position or the pressure of
holding the stance will detract from the meditation. The Tai Chi
Standing Posts could be used, as could any posture drawn from
Shibashi, Tao Yin, Lotus, or Lohan.

CHI MEDITATION FOR THE MICROCOSMIC ORBIT

We are going to start our chi meditation by working on the main energy
circuit of the body. This is the circuit formed by the connection of the
du mai (governing vessel) and *ren mai* (conception vessel).

There are two ways the chi energy can be "encouraged" to flow
within this circuit. The first is by focusing mentally on acupoints on the
du mai and *ren mai* meridians in sequence; the second is to imagine
moving a small sphere of energy along the path of the meridians. It is
also possible to combine these techniques. If you have difficulty holding
a visualization, you can start off by actually placing the fingertips over
the acupoint being visualized. (This becomes impossible later on, unless
you are a contortionist!)

The second technique used is to imagine a small sphere of energy,
about the size and appearance of a gold-colored golf ball, at the
location of each acupoint. The acupoints should be visualized as being
about an inch inside the body.

How to open up acupoints

The first time that you visualize each acupoint, you should maintain the
visualization of the energy sphere at the acupoint location, about one
inch inside the body, for about five minutes. Be very aware of any
physical changes, such as warmth, you may feel in the area. Do not be
concerned if you feel the urge to wriggle or jerk; this is quite normal

when energy blockages are dispersed. Any such symptoms should gradually diminish over time.

When you first start the meditation, you may find your concentration is limited. Do not worry about this. Even if you only succeed in focusing on one point in early sessions, you are making progress.

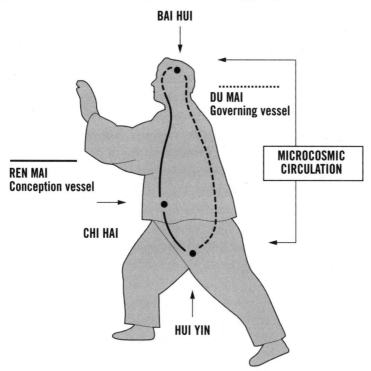

You must always start your chi meditation at the *tan tien* (*shenque* CV 8, see table on page 66), moving downwards along the *ren mai* and upwards along the *du mai*. You must open up each acupoint in sequence. Once you have opened up an acupoint, you may reduce the meditation time on the acupoint to one minute and then proceed to the next point.

When you become tired, or run out of time, slowly bring your point of focus back along the meridians to the *tan tien* and concentrate on that area for a minute or two. Always re-center your energy at *tan tien* — this is most important.

Should you encounter unpleasant or disturbing sensations during your meditation practice, re-center your energy at *tan tien*. If the symptoms are particularly disturbing, or do not diminish with practice, cease, and seek advice from a person trained in chi meditation.

It is obvious from the above description and the number of points to be opened up in the microcosmic orbit that it is probably going to take you six or more meditation sessions to open up all the points. Do not be in any hurry.

When we talk about moving the point of awareness, or the visualization of the sphere, this should be done slowly and evenly. Imagine a ping-pong ball either slowly sinking or floating up through honey and you will have the correct imagery. Each time you have either opened up or focused on an acupoint, move the sphere along the meridian to the next point or return it to the tan tien.

ACUPOINTS ON WHICH TO MEDITATE IN THE MICROCOSMIC ORBIT

CV 8	*Shenque*	Immediately behind the navel
CV 6	*Chi hai*	Three finger-widths below the navel
CV 4	*Guan yuan*	Two finger-widths above the pubic bone
CV 2	*Qugu*	At the upper border of the pubic bone
CV 1	*Hui yin*	In the center of the perineum (between the anus and the genitals)
GV 2	*Yao shu*	One inch up from the tip of the coccyx (tail bone), in the hiatus of the sacrum
GV 4	*Ming men*	Between the first and second lumbar vertebrae
GV 6	*Zi zhong*	Between the eleventh and twelfth thoracic vertebrae
GV 16	*Feng fu*	At the base of the skull
GV 20	*Bai hui*	At the midpoint of the line connecting the apex of the ears
	Yin tang	At the mid-point between the eyebrows
GV 25	*Su liao*	At the tip of the nose
CV 22	*Tian tu*	In the notch of the bones at the base of the throat (technically the center of the suprasternal fossa)
CV 17	*Dan zhong*	In men, located between the nipples. In women, a little over an inch from the base of the sternum, technically on a level with the fourth intercostal space
CV 12	*Zhong wan*	Four finger-widths above the umbilicus

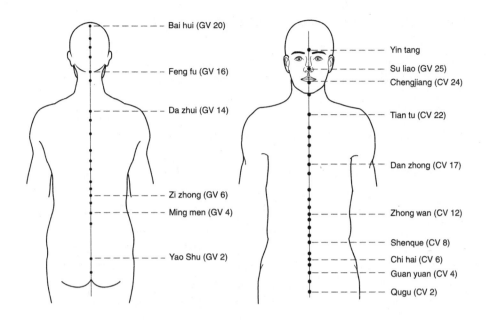

It is impracticable to focus on all the points located on the governing and conception vessels. As there are fifty-two of them, it is the points with major impact on the body's energy flows which have been selected for this meditation. The movement of the point of visualization along the meridians will effectively open up all of the remaining points.

Remember to re-center your energy.

Chi meditation for the macrocosmic orbit

When you are comfortable with the microcosmic orbit, you can begin to open up the macrocosmic orbit. Whereas the former involves only the torso and head, the latter involves all of the limbs as well. One can either meditate on the points in the legs and the arms simultaneously, or treat each limb separately, one after the other.

ACUPOINTS ON WHICH TO FOCUS IN THE MACROCOSMIC ORBIT

CV 8	*Shenque*	Immediately behind the navel
CV 1	*Hui yin*	In the center of the perineum (between the anus and the genitals)
BL 40	*Wei zhong*	At the center of the back of the knees
KI 1	*Yong quan*	At the soles of the feet in the junction of the anterior (front)/middle sole
SP 1	*Yin bai*	On the big toe just below the bottom of the toenail root
SP 2	*Da du*	Extends along the inside edge of the foot to the joint of the lower bone of the toe
	He dig	At the top of the knee
GV 4	*Ming men*	Between the first and second lumbar vertebrae
GV 14	*Da zhui*	Between the spinous process of the seventh cervical vertebrae and the first thoracic vertebrae
LI 11	*Qu chi*	On the outside end of the elbow crease when the arm is flexed
PC 8	*Lao gong*	At the center of the palm
TJ 5	*Wai guan*	At the back of the wrist, three finger-widths from the crease
GV 20	*Bai hui*	At the midpoint of the line connecting the apex of the ears
CV 17	*Dan zhong*	In men, located between the nipples. In women, a little over an inch from the base of the sternum, technically on a level with the fourth intercostal space

Remember to re-center your energy.

HEALTH BENEFITS

Chi underlies all physical and mental activities. Improving the chi flow through the application of chi meditation techniques may therefore have the following general positive effects on the body and mind: increased relaxation, and improved circulation and functioning of organ systems; you should be in a more optimistic frame of mind; your emotional balance should improve; and there should be a general increase in your ability to concentrate and to learn and retain facts.

Chi meditation techniques involve good posture and breathing, and these will also have positive effects on the body and mind. If you are suffering adverse symptoms from chi blockage or poor chi circulation, these symptoms should be alleviated or disappear.

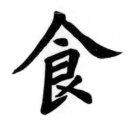

Chapter Six

Chi Diet

WHAT IS THE CHI DIET?

THE CHI DIET IS AN APPROACH to nutrition which developed in China over thousands of years, its overall objective being a long and healthy life. The chi diet seeks to maintain one's health and energy and to prevent the onset of disease. It needs to be distinguished from Chinese food medicine, which deals with the use of food to cure diseases and infections which have already established themselves within the body.

The chi diet recognizes that the nutritional needs of an individual will vary, depending on his or her age, constitution, and occupation. The chi diet also varies according to environment and season. Rather than providing lists of foods and the quantities and proportions in which they should be eaten, the chi diet seeks to provide each individual with the skills and knowledge necessary to ensure his or her diet provides an adequate supply of chi. It is as much about how we eat, as what we eat.

One of the first things to realize is that following a chi diet does not necessitate consumption of Chinese food. This confuses Chinese cuisine with Chinese dietary theory. The first refers to the type of meals the Chinese like to cook and consume; the second to a body of principles that can be applied to the consumption of any food.

Naturally, some foods and combinations of foods are more healthy than others, but what we eat is not always a matter of choice. There are often other considerations such as:

- availability of food types;
- relative costs;
- ethical and religious considerations; and
- social custom.

The theory of the chi diet deals not only with what the best foods are for an individual at a particular period of time but sets out the general principles of how to mix, prepare, and eat the foods.

The chi diet is guided by principles, according to which these nutritional techniques can be varied to suit individual needs and make the best of the foods available. The theory supplements, rather than replaces, other nutritional theories.

In the Chinese mind, eating and health are intimately related, yet such a relationship does not detract from the enjoyment derived from eating Chinese food. In fact, Chinese cuisine is generally recognized as one of the truly great cuisines of the world. The proper application of the chi diet can give you the best of both worlds: healthy yet stimulating eating.

CHI AND NUTRITION

In the West, the science of nutrition concerns itself primarily with the quantity and respective proportions that we should consume of the five major nutrients found in foods — proteins, fats, starches, sugars, and acids — along with vitamins, minerals, and dietary fiber.

This knowledge is certainly important for a healthy diet. It does, however, reflect the West's focus on the physical rather than the energetic, on calorie intake and the caloric values of food; in essence, a physical approach that determines how much "fuel" you need to take on board.

To see the limitations of such an approach, you might apply it to putting gasoline into a car. We know that some cars run better on super and some on regular gasoline, and that it is not a good idea to run any car on aviation fuel! If we applied this "calorie concept" to gasoline, buying it by the calorie and ignoring the strength and concentration of energy in the fuel, we would have a lot of motor vehicles with damaged engines! Clearly, we need to take a more sophisticated approach to the energy side of the food equation.

The Chinese perceive all matter to be a reflection of an underlying energy pattern. This energy pattern is its chi.

What the Chinese sought to do in a chi diet was to identify the underlying nature of the energy pattern within each type of food. Once this energy pattern was identified, by applying the theories of yin and yang and the five elements one could predict the effect of the energy pattern of the food on an individual. One could then look at the constitution, age, and occupation of the individual and, taking into account his or her local environment and the season, recommend particular quantities and proportions of foods. Interestingly, long before the Chinese knew anything of vitamins, proteins, carbohydrates, or fats, they had evolved diets consistent with that which modern Western science would now recommend as healthy.

In fact, Chinese dietary concepts include areas only recently touched on by Western nutritional science, such as the hazards and benefits of combining certain types of foods at one meal. This was only raised in the West in the 1920s.

Such Chinese dietary successes were achieved through the development of the theories of the "five flavors" and "five energies" of food. These theories are built on three underlying concepts which are consistent throughout Chinese health theory:

- chi theory;
- yin/yang theory; and
- five elements (or five elemental energies) theory.

To summarize, the Chinese sought to look at food from the perspective of how it influenced the energy (or chi) balance within the individual. The idea was that when various food "structures" are taken into the body, the ensuing breaking down of them releases the chi related to that structure, making it available for incorporation into the body. The chi released can vary, both as to its quantity and nature.

When examined in terms of its effect on a person, the nature of food chi has three main aspects:

- The degree to which it is perceived as having a "heating" or "cooling" effect on the human body. This is the "five energies" effect.
- The "drying" or "moistening" effect of the food on the body.
- The affinity and effect that the food chi has on a particular organ system. (This may be predicted from the "five taste theory" detailed later, which is one aspect of the five elemental energies theory.)

ELEMENTS OF THE NUTRITION PROCESS

As discussed, in the West the key aspects of nutrition theory, as understood by the general public, involve ingesting what is deemed to be the appropriate quantity of fats, carbohydrates, proteins, vitamins, and trace elements, with such quantities being based largely on the rate of calorie expenditure and the deemed correct weight of the body for its age, sex, and height.

Of course, nutritionists will consider other matters as well but only a small percentage of Westerners have the benefit of such advice. For many, a person's diet is perceived to be healthy if it keeps him or her the "right" shape. That it might also predispose the person to illness, depression, and lethargy is often a secondary consideration.

How and where you eat, and that eating should be an enjoyable activity, seem to be dismissed as nutritional considerations; in fact, enjoyment of food is often considered incompatible with good nutrition. However, these considerations are, of course, very important factors in the chi diet.

The first step to take in the chi diet is the same as that taken in the Western approach to nutrition, but it is from a different perspective. That is, while each approach involves an analysis of what a person needs from his or her diet, the Chinese focus is on the total effect of the diet on body, mind, emotions, and spirit via the energetic system, while the Western focus is on bodily needs and the metabolic effect of a diet.

In the Western approach, once dietary needs have been determined a person simply acquires and ingests the required amount of the specified foods. In the Chinese approach, the determination of dietary needs is only the starting point. There are a number of processes between the point of harvest and the point of digestion that can enhance, degrade, or simply change the nature and quantity of the chi in food. To maximize the benefits of your diet, it is most important to ensure that all the following processes take place in the most beneficial way:

- Maximizing the quantity of chi in the actual food at the point of purchase or collection.
- Maintaining, enhancing, or changing the nature and quantity of the food chi during any storage or preservative process that takes place between the time of acquisition and the time of consumption.
- Maintaining, enhancing, or changing the nature and

quantity of the food chi during the cooking and preparation process.

- Maintaining or enhancing the quantity of food chi through the consumption process.
- Maintaining or enhancing the quantity of food chi through the digestion process.

Each of these processes is examined in detail later in this section.

The Chinese approach in determining which foods (and what quantities of it) are required by an individual is so different from the Western one that we must first examine how the Chinese view food, its purpose and effects. This will require a review of some of your current beliefs about food.

CHINESE DIETARY THEORY

"To eat or not to eat" — that seems to be the question!

If you have read much about diet and nutrition you may be somewhat confused by the contradictory nature of many of the opinions expressed. Everybody seems to have a personal barrow to push. What possible purpose, you might think, is there in looking at yet another approach to nutrition, that will probably make following a good diet even harder! You may have heard, for instance, that:

- You should not eat the meat of birds, animals, or fish for ethical reasons, or because of health problems caused by humans "not having evolved" to digest meat.
- You should not eat dairy products, such as milk, cheese, and yogurt, because they are unhealthy.
- You should not eat any fruits or vegetables not grown locally, out of season, or on which pesticides and fertilizers have been used.
- You should not eat grain foods, as they are not part of our natural diet and have to be processed before becoming digestible.
- You should not eat any processed food, any food with additives, or any food subjected to pasteurization, sterilization, irradiation, genetic engineering, etc.
- You should not eat raw foods because the proteins

within them are difficult to digest and may contain
hostile bacteria and organisms.
- You should not eat cooked foods because cooking
reduces the protein quality and nutritional value is lost.

While, individually, there may be sound reasoning behind each of
these statements, when taken together they do not leave you many
dietary options. Basically, if you complied with all these strictures you
would have to survive on such local nuts, fruits, berries, and fungi you
could find growing wild. If people took the above too seriously, the
result would be:
- Mass starvation, with the death of perhaps 90 percent of
people currently alive.
- The total disbanding of all technology and agriculture,
including those elements promoting sanitation and
hygiene, resulting in a massive increase in disease and
infection.
- The reversion to an existence where people spent 90 percent of their waking time collecting food and where a
drought, fire, pest infestation, or flood meant probable
starvation.

These are somewhat high prices to pay for a "healthy" diet!

Of course, the advocates of such measures do not want the results
described above. Instead, they believe that they and their followers
should live in the "healthy" way, while the rest of society provides the
positive "benefits" of a technological civilization. However, when a
whole society follows certain ways of living (rather than a limited
number of individuals in a society), this impacts strongly on the whole
way of life of that society's members.

Thus, while a diet of wild nuts, fruits, and berries may have a high
nutritional health value, the associated lifestyle choices that go with
such a diet may have health negatives far outweighing the benefits
conferred by it. It can easily be shown from an examination of the
remains of individuals who were members of ancient hunter-gatherer
societies that members of these societies lived far shorter, more
unhealthy lives than we do now, even with all our dietary problems!

The message here, though, is not that we should be complacent about
our current diets. Indeed, far from it! In our case, the evolution of an
industrial society brought certain approaches to nutrition that need a

long hard rethink. However, a "purist" approach to diet is simply not practicable. As in all things, there must be compromise.

The chi diet teaches you how to make the best of the food options currently available to you and how to get the most out of your current diet. It should do this whether you are a strict vegetarian or an ardent meat eater; and whether you carefully plan your diet or subsist largely on junk food. It cannot eliminate damage caused by a poor diet but it can reduce and make the most of whatever benefits can be derived from the food.

Other influences on diet

People's dietary habits often involve considerations besides nutrition. Two of the thorniest issues involve the consumption of animals and alcohol. (I would point out that the discussion in this book is from a chi perspective only and no religious, moral, or ethical judgments are made or intended — these are something an individual has to resolve personally.)

Vegetarianism

While some regions in China were influenced by Buddhist thought, the Chinese have generally consumed meat and seafood. However, even where religious and moral beliefs have not impinged on the consumption of meat, there has always been a general belief that the consumption of large quantities of it should be avoided.

For instance, Zhu Danxi (1281–1385), a medical scientist in the Yuan Dynasty, advised in his work *Ru dan Lun* (Benefits of Plain Food on Health) following a mainly vegetarian diet, eating meat and vegetables in appropriate proportions. He advocated eating mainly grains, beans, vegetables, and fruit and a limited amount of meat, cautioning that one should not eat more meat than vegetables. *The Mystery of Longevity* by Liu Zhengcai states that eating too much meat regularly impairs the health and shortens life.

While believing that the moral or ethical aspects of eating meats are a matter for the individual to decide, it is objectionable that some advocates use facts selectively to establish a scientific basis for their beliefs.

One example is the argument that humans are not evolved to eat meat. It is not the lack of acknowledgment of the fact that our digestive systems have evolved enzymes in order to digest meat that is disturbing so much as people not being told that some individuals may pay a price in terms of their health and well-being if they attempt to become vegetarians.

Daniel Reid points out in *The Tao of Health, Sex and Longevity* that while we first evolved as herbivores we have also adapted to consume meat, and this includes the way in which our metabolism works. According to Reid, the human race seems to have "hedged its bets" in this evolution, with about 25 percent of people having metabolisms mainly suited to a vegetarian diet, 25 percent being suited to a meat-based diet, and about 50 percent having metabolisms that can cope reasonably well with both diets.

Reid suggests that you can easily determine your own metabolic type by consuming a steak or a piece of chicken. If you feel exhausted and lethargic afterwards, you may well have a system that would be more comfortable with a vegetarian diet. If you feel strong, vital, and mentally alert, you need a meat-based diet.

It would probably be helpful to see if reducing the quantity of meat you eat improves your health. *The Yellow Emperor's Classic of Internal Medicine* states: "The quantity of meats should not exceed that of other foodstuffs."

Consumption of alcohol

Alcohol has caused many social problems in China and elsewhere. Liu Zhengcai notes in *The Mystery of Longevity* that *Lu's Almanac* (*Lu Shi Chun Qui*) says that heavy drinking is significant in the incidence of disease. However, he goes on to say that drinking a limited amount of liquor is beneficial. This is based on the following facts:

- Fermented drinks, such as beer or wine, are the only drinks which assist the digestive process.
- The "circulatory boost" given by alcohol can be very beneficial for older people.
- Red wines are a good source of anti-oxidants.
- Alcohol is also used to "carry" energy in other foods and herbs, and is used in Chinese traditional medicine in tonics. (Much the same situation exists in the West, where even persons vigorously opposed to drinking alcohol in wines, beers, and spirits cheerfully resort to cough medicines and tonics which, more often than not, are largely alcohol-based.)

Recent Western studies found that groups of people who drank small amounts of alcohol tended to live longer than control groups who did not drink any. Groups of people who drank large amounts of alcohol, however, severely shortened their life expectancies.

Perhaps Hsuechui, an imperial physician of the Yuan Dynasty, sums the situation up best in *Essentials of Food and Drink* (*Yin Shan Zheng Yao*):

> Liquor ... brings the function of medicinal herbs into full play in the human body, eliminates all evils, promotes blood circulation, nourishes stomach and intestines and dissipates worries. Therefore, if one drinks a limited amount of liquor, it keeps him in good health. Excessive drinking impairs the mind, shortens the life span and changes one's intrinsic nature.

It seems, then, that liquor should be thought of as a powerful medicine to be used with caution.

The Chinese view of the role of food

In China there is much less distinction between daily food consumption and the application of preventative and corrective health regimes than there is in the West. In China, eating is believed to maintain a correct individual energy balance and is thus primarily preventative in nature (though it has a major secondary role as an energy balance cure). When a person's sense of well-being is not what it should be, or when sickness strikes, the Chinese inclination is to look at modifying his or her diet; and there are many more "food cures" in China, both in traditional Chinese folklore and in the armory of formal health practitioners, than in the West.

It is only necessary to draw on a selection of historical and literary references to demonstrate the long-term connection that the Chinese have made between eating and health. Chinese concerns about food can be traced back millennia, as can be seen from the following:

- *The Yellow Emperor's Classic of Internal Medicine* enjoins its readers to: "Eat and drink moderately and adjust the various food types and flavors to the seasons and one's state of health."
- During the Chou Dynasty the imperial government was

said to have appointed officials whose job it was to plan the diet of the imperial household, so that meals provided adequate nourishment, did not consist of foods that clashed, and were adjusted according to seasonal changes.

- Confucius devoted a whole chapter of his *Analects* to various techniques that should be followed when eating.
- Zhang Zhonjing, during the Eastern Han Dynasty, wrote in *Synopsis of the Golden Chamber*:

  Food and drink are beneficial to health but only when taken appropriately, both as to quality and quantity; otherwise they can become detrimental. Moreover, for sick persons, suitable food will be beneficial to the recovery from illness, whilst unsuitable food aggravates the condition.

- Zhang Hua (265–420 AD) wrote that: "The less one eats, the broader one's mind and the longer one's lifespan. The more one eats, the narrower one's mind and the shorter one's lifespan."
- In the sixth century AD Sun Shu Mao wrote in *One Thousand Gold Remedies for Emergencies* that: "A true doctor first finds out the cause of a disease and, having found that out, tries to cure it first by food."
- In 1307 Cou Xuan wrote:

  Physicians must recognize the causes of an illness and know what transgression of the normal regular balance of yin and yang has taken place. To correct this imbalance, adequate diet is the first necessity. Only when this has failed should drugs be prescribed.

- Around 1330 the imperial physician of the Mongol court wrote:

  Therefore, he who would nourish his nature should eat only when he is hungry and not fill himself with food; he should drink only when he is thirsty and not fill himself with drink; he should eat little and between long intervals and not too much and not too constantly; he should aim at being a little hungry when filled and being a little well-filled when hungry.

Being well-filled hurts the lungs and being hungry hurts the flow of vital energy.
- In 1368 Chia Ming wrote in the *Essential Knowledge for Eating and Drinking*:

  Food and drink are relied on to nurture life. But if one does not know that the nature of substances may be opposed to each other and one consumes them together indiscriminately, the vital organs will be thrown out of harmony and disastrous consequences will soon arise. Therefore, those who wish to nurture their lives must carefully avoid doing such damage to themselves.
- Gong Tingxian, the imperial physician of the Ming Dynasty, wrote: "Eat to be only half full and of no more than two dishes. Drink seldom and then only three tenths of one's capacity."

Food for body, mind, and spirit

It is important to note that when, as in China, food is spoken of as the "first resource" which should be used to correct an energy imbalance, you should not think only of energy imbalances reflected as physical symptoms. Food is also the first resource in curing emotional, mental, and spiritual imbalances.

The Chinese explanation of how the chi in food affects our mental and physical states can be found in the theory of the five elemental energies: see page 82. It should also be emphasized that Chinese theories of diet aim to prevent problems rather than correct them. Thus, in determining your diet you should also look at, for example:
- the season;
- your age;
- your activities; and
- your environment.

As these change, there is a need for you to make dietary adjustments just to maintain your balanced energy state.

Herbs and the "forgotten foods"

As mentioned, Chinese nutritional principles primarily aim to be preventative by ensuring against energy imbalances, on the basis that such imbalances will, sooner or later, be reflected as sickness in the body, mind, and spirit. Thus, the principles are intended first to prevent an energy imbalance and, if this fails, at least to correct it before sickness can ensue.

When sickness does occur, more dramatic action must be taken, generally through the use of herbs and "forgotten foods." (Such action, while based on the principles we have examined, tends to involve detailed, specialist knowledge.)

THE CHI DIET AND ASSESSING INDIVIDUAL DIETARY NEEDS

Because of the underlying concept of matching individual nutrition to individual energy, or chi needs, there is no "official" Chinese chi diet, and one should be wary of any diet that calls itself Chinese-based and prescribes one diet for all. Rather, in a Chinese chi diet, an individual's diet must be tailored to his or her individual energy condition.

This is fine if you are preparing meals only for yourself but presents more difficulty if you are preparing meals for a number of people who may have widely different food needs.

Practically speaking, one or two meals are not likely to have much impact on your health. It is your long-term diet which is important and, on this basis, you need to ensure the long-term dietary needs of you and your children are met as best as possible.

It is interesting that the Chinese concept of banquet-type meals (consisting of many small dishes) for larger and more formal occasions may have gained popularity and acceptance because it allows participants to make selections that meet their individual dietary needs.

On a day-to-day basis, in the past the individual could assess his or her own dietary needs either by seeing the local health advisor or, as was more likely, by performing a personal assessment of his or her energy needs. This was liable to be informal but could be done by, for example, the *si jian* (four examinations): see Chapter 7. Whether informal or not, such an examination basically involved assessment of overall yin/yang balance at the organ system level.

Diet, and the relative ways in which food could correct energy imbalances and alleviate symptoms, was, and is, a general subject for discussion amongst members of the Chinese community at a social level. There would be nothing unusual about a self-assessment of dietary needs being quite detailed and sophisticated. This is one area where positive changes could be made to the Western approach.

After deciding what energy imbalances you have, or are likely to incur, the next question is: how can you tell whether a particular food will correct or aggravate a particular condition? The answer to this lies in the application of the "five energies theory" and the "five tastes theory."

The five energies

The Chinese place foods into five categories, each with a yin/yang effect on the energy balance of the body:

- hot: extreme yang;
- warming: slightly yang;
- neutral: balance of yin and yang;
- cooling: slightly yin; and
- cold: extreme yin.

It is important to remember that these descriptions do not relate to the temperature of the food at the time of ingestion but to the effect that it has on the body's energy system. For instance, putting chillies in the fridge will not significantly change the yang effect they have on your body. (A possible exception to this is the effect of neutral foods, which may be influenced by their temperature.) Thus, despite the fact they are served hot, the teas drunk in the West have a predominantly cooling effect; alcohol, despite the fact that it is most often served cold, has a predominantly heating effect.

Another thing to note with these yin/yang categorizations is that just because there are five energy measures, this does not mean you should try to relate them to the five elements theory (five elemental energies: see page 83). The five elements theory deals with the nature, rather than magnitude, of energy effect.

The various energy ratings given to different foods are arrived at solely from experience. There are many tables available, showing common foods and which energy categories they fall into, but you do not have to rely on other people's judgment or carry food tables around. Simply eat a food and make your own assessment of what effect it has had on your body. That is, how do you feel? Hot, as after chili peppers? Cool, as after cucumber? You should make this judgment about ten minutes after finishing the food, so as to eliminate the purely transitional effect that derives from the temperature of the food ingested.

The five tastes

The other theory which allows us to predict a food's effect is the five elements theory. This states that the five elemental energies — wood, fire, earth, metal, and water — are associated with a specific taste.

TASTE	ELEMENTAL ENERGY	ASSOCIATED ORGAN SYSTEMS	FOOD EXAMPLE
SOUR	WOOD	LIVER and cleansing systems. Sour foods solidify the contents of the digestive tract.	LEMON
BITTER	FIRE	HEART and circulatory system. Bitter foods dry the system and purge the bowels.	HOPS
SWEET	EARTH	SPLEEN and digestive system. Sweet foods disperse stagnant energy, promote circulation, and harmonize the stomach.	HONEY
PUNGENT OR SPICY	METAL	LUNGS and respiratory system. Spicy foods disperse accumulated toxins.	GINGER
SALTY	WATER	KIDNEY and eliminative systems. Salty foods soften and moisten tissues and facilitate bowel movements.	SEAWEED

HOW TO MAXIMIZE CHI THROUGH THE FIVE NUTRITION PROCESSES

The previous sections have provided the basis for determining which foods you need to include in your overall diet. Now we will examine the five nutrition processes.

Assessing and selecting food

The first process involves maximizing the quantity of the chi in food at the point of purchase or collection.

When people evolved as hunter-gatherers they did not have to worry about how the food they had hunted or gathered had been grown or raised, since each plant and animal had grown in its own way. Rather, the problem was finding and catching food on a regular enough basis to satisfy the hunger of the family group.

The introduction of agriculture and the domestication of animals largely solved the food quantity problems faced by the hunter-gatherer societies. However, there was a trade-off. The negative aspects of the trade-off were as follows:

- People tended to reduce the variety of their diets. Only plants that could be grown easily or animals that could be domesticated easily formed part of the new diets.
- Quality became a problem. The growing of foods in unnatural locations and the keeping of animals in unnatural habitats impacted on the quantity of the chi that could be obtained from the food. There is some belief that the nature of the particular chi may change if there is a dramatic alteration in the lifestyle, diet, and physical structure of a plant or animal. Certainly, any change in its category or degree of taste would have to be taken as indication of such an energy change. (This "quality" deterioration has only increased as technology and food production methods have developed, with various hormones and antibiotics being added to food to increase the efficiency of production.)

It should be emphasized that while the trade-off had negative aspects, it still represented a great leap forward for most of humankind. That is:

- length of life increased;
- human societies grew larger and more complex; and
- there was increased opportunity for mental, physical, and spiritual development.

(It is true that some significant hunter–gatherer civilizations, such as the Australian Aborigines, have been severely damaged by exposure to modern industrial societies, but this damage does not seem to relate primarily to the change in food consumption patterns.)

Whatever we think of the various agricultural and industrial revolutions which have taken place, it is how we deal with the negative effects of these revolutions that affects our lives. The following suggestions are for the purpose of improving the quantity of the chi in the foods we all eat. Remember that if you can satisfy all the requirements, you are doing very well.

When possible, choose fruits and plants in the following order of preference:

1. **Organically grown:** That is, without pesticides and artificially produced chemical stimulants.
2. **In season:** This has two aspects: first, the nature of the chi is appropriate; and, second, there has been less opportunity for deterioration and the use of preservative processes. (Sun drying, for preservation, and storage in dry, dark, cool locations may sometimes improve chi.)
3. **Healthy looking:** For healthy read natural, not the artificially enhanced colors which can often be found, for example, in apples and egg yolks.
4. **Locally grown:** If grown locally (and in season) the nature of chi associated with the food should be "in tune" with the chi of the local environment and is more likely to meet the body's needs. If foods are not grown locally, select foods from an environment with the same seasonal conditions.

When possible, choose meats, poultry, and fish in the following order of preference:

1. **Animals raised in the wild**
2. **Domesticated animals:** That is, those that have had a life and a diet as close as possible to what they would have experienced in the wild and which are free of hormones and antibiotics, for example, free-range chickens. Avoid fish, fowl, and meat products produced on an "intensive" basis.
3. **Healthy looking:** For healthy read natural, not the artificially enhanced colors which can often be found in, for example, meats laced with monosodium glutomate.
4. **Locally raised:** If raised locally (and in season) the nature of chi associated with the animals should be "in tune" with the chi of the local environment and is more likely to meet the body's needs. If animals are not raised locally, select them from an environment with the same seasonal conditions.

Storing, transporting, and preserving food

The second process involves maintaining, enhancing, or changing the nature and quantity of the food chi during any storage or preservative process that takes place between the time of acquisition and the time of consumption.

That is, the effect on nature and quality of food that may be caused by:

- the manner in which the food item was harvested, transported, and stored;
- the length of time between the harvesting and consumption of the food; and
- the methods used to "preserve" the food during the delay between harvesting and consumption.

In most cases, you will not know how a food item has been harvested, transported, or stored and will have to rely on its appearance to guess the conditions to which it has been subjected. Look out for signs of bruising, loss of color, excessive dryness, or moistness.

If you are harvesting, transporting, or storing the food yourself, try to avoid doing any of this in excessive heat or damp, as these accelerate the degenerative effect. The obvious exceptions are moist foods, which should be kept moist, preferably by being kept in a sealed environment. Obviously, the food should be subjected to as little physical damage as possible.

Foods that are to be stored should generally be placed in cool, dry, dark areas (the exceptions being moist foods, which should not be allowed to dehydrate).

As can be seen from the above, it is virtually impossible to talk about the transportation and storage of food without raising preservation of food. This can be as non-invasive as storage in a cool, dry place, or involve the full gamut of chemical preservation and radiation.

There are many methods of preserving foods, including sun drying, smoking, salting, pickling, sealing, freezing, irradiating, and chemically preserving. Each preservative process has a specific effect on the quantity and nature of the chi inside the food, while not necessarily simply being destructive of chi quantity. For instance:

- Sun drying, dehydration, and smoking can concentrate the chi.
- Pickling and salting can change the nature of the chi.

This is neither good nor bad in itself; it depends on what you want the nature of the chi to be, which in turn depends on your individual needs.

- Freezing seems, at best, a neutral process that can slow chi loss.
- Chemical preservatives should not be opposed simply because they are artificial but because how they will affect chi is unknown. Any substance ingested can affect the body's chi.
- The jury is still out on irradiation. It is not an additive, and some of the current responses may simply be emotional, coming from people who may have opposed the discovery of fire if they had been around at the time!

Preservative processes are also a potential solution to the problem posed by an old Chinese adage that you should not eat a food unless it rots but that you should not eat it when it rots. The concept here is that if a food does not rot, either its chi structure is so stable that living organisms cannot break it down or it is so "unhealthy" that no other organism will touch it. Either way, it is not likely to do the human organism much good!

With the exception of some foods which have undergone preservation processes such as pickling and fermentation, the fresher the food, the better. So buy small amounts of food frequently, rather than buying large amounts and storing them.

Cooking and preparing food

The third process involves maintaining, enhancing, or changing the nature and quantity of the food chi during the cooking, meal design, and food presentation process.

This process basically concerns the creation of a meal. While the Western approach is to look at the overall diet, little attention is paid to the individual meal in its own right. Yet, it is at the meal stage that many important factors come into play. For instance, the Chinese say that food should have the following qualities, being:

- pleasing in aroma;
- pleasing in taste;
- pleasing to the eyes; and
- pleasing to the body.

There are two questions that must be answered before we look at the specific aspects of cooking, meal design, and food presentation:

- Why do these qualities matter? Just dump the food in a heap on the plate. It may not look or smell good but it will be just as healthy!
- What if you have gone to all the trouble of finding out what your body, mind, emotions, and spirit need and the required foods just don't have those qualities?

No one would deny that having an argument in the middle of a meal, or worrying during a meal, lessens its benefits. Such things are known to have a dramatic impact on the digestive process, particularly the ability to produce the required digestive juices. The Chinese take this one step further, believing that the more the senses are pleasantly stimulated, the more favorable your impressions of the meal will be and the more effective will be the absorption of chi into your body. If the food is repulsive-looking, smelly slop, then your focus on it will be negative and this will interfere with chi absorption.

While your diet must be balanced, there is no particular reason why an individual meal should be balanced. In fact, since our bodies' digestive systems must cope with different foods in distinct, often opposed, ways, the concept of having a little of everything at each meal is a most unhealthy one.

Limiting the number of food types does not mean that you have to limit the number of food tastes. Rather than having, say, three dinners on consecutive days, each made up of one type of meat, one type of green vegetable, and one type of carbohydrate (potato and/or bread), it would be much better to have one meal of mixed meats, one meal of mixed vegetables, and one meal of mixed carbohydrates. The overall dietary intake is exactly the same, but the likelihood of digestive problems is reduced and the possibility of making each meal quite different from the preceding one is enhanced.

At any individual meal it is possible to supplement "required" foods with those which are not, as long as they are consumed in a quantity and manner that does not adversely affect the overall diet. Such supplementary foods can be balanced so that their opposite effects cancel each other out, having a neutral effect on your energy balance.

There are many methods of cooking, preparing, and presenting food, and these techniques influence both the quantity and the nature of chi.

Some combinations of food energies are beneficial, while others are not. The proportions of foods should not be ignored, and neither should the effect of various spices, salts, sauces, and herbs.

Cooking

The advent of the discovery of fire lead to the possibility of "cooking" food. This was a major advance. Cai Jingeng in *Eating your Way to Health — Dietotherapy in Traditional Chinese Medicine*, says that cooked food increases the body's resistance to disease because its nutrients are more easily digested than those in raw food.

Cooking is so significant in "preparing" food that the two terms have virtually come to mean the same thing, with cooks now preparing our salads! In this book, however, we shall preserve the distinction, and the word "cook" or "cooking" should be taken to involve the application of heat.

The "art" of cooking provides some of the best evidence that there is "something" (chi) involved in cooking that makes it more than a chemical process. Who would want to eat a meal prepared by someone who believed that there was no difference between cooking and chemistry, and that all that was required was the transfer of thermal heat energy into a food substance to provoke certain chemical reactions? Unfortunately, one may suspect this is all too frequently the perception of the food technologists who design and prepare much of the preprocessed food we eat today.

The myriad effects that we can achieve by cooking the same food, depending on whether the heat applied is that of an open flame, gas, electricity, charcoal, etc.; the distance the food is from the heat source; the nature and shape of any material between the heat source and the food, such as a griddle, hotplate, saucepan, etc.; and the nature of movement that the food undergoes while in the presence of the heat source simply cannot be explained by saying that cooking is all to do with the amount of thermal energy absorbed over a given period of time.

There is a further advantage of cooking: the opportunity to eat food at a temperature less than or equal to body temperature. There is little advantage, and considerable danger, in ingesting food that is hotter than body temperature. The stomach is designed to carry out its digestive functions best at body temperature.

When food is at a temperature lower than body temperature, digestion slows until the food heats up. This means that peristalsis may take the food into areas not designed to receive partially digested food. It also means that heat will flow from the core of the body to the stomach, and lowering of core body temperature can interfere with metabolic functions and predispose the body to infection and illness.

The Chinese believe that the most beneficial method of eating is to eat a broth or soup at body temperature. This is particularly important where the body is in a weakened state from illness, injury, or old age. (Interestingly, these are just the types of situations where soups and broths would be served in the West.)

Lin Yutang, a noted Chinese philosopher, stated:
> Chinese medicines are often served as stews and called soups. It is made like an ordinary soup, in that it must be made with the proper regard for the mixing of flavor and ingredients. The stew is designed not just to attack the illness but to nourish and strengthen the body as a whole.

An ancient Chinese proverb also notes:
> SOUPS — First, drink soup when eating a meal, so that in old age the body will not be harmed.

One further consideration is whether cooking results in loss of nutritional value. Bob Flaws, an expert in traditional Chinese medicine, uses the following example in dealing with this problem. Flaws notes that the critical aspect of nutrition, in so far as the body is concerned, is not the nutritional value of the food ingested (taken into the digestive system) but the nutritional value assimilated into the body, less the energy costs of such assimilation.

Thus, an item of food may have 100 nutritional units in its raw state but, due to its raw state, digestion will only be 75 percent and the energy expended by the body in assimilating the food might be a further ten nutritional units. On this basis, the body has a net gain of sixty-five nutritional units.

Raw: 100 NU – 25 (lost in digestion) – 10 (energy expended) = 65 NU gain

If the food is cooked, digestion might rise to 85 percent and energy expended fall to five units. In this case, the net energy gain is eighty nutritional units.

Cooked: 100 NU − 15 (lost in digestion) − 5 (energy expended) = 80 NU gain

Thus, apart from the other benefits of cooking, the net nutritional gain to the consumer may be increased through the cooking process.

Meal design

It should immediately be realized that there is a significant difference between meal design and diet design. There are many foods which should be a part of your diet that should not be present in one meal at one time. The energies are incompatible and so are the chemical reactions that may occur (or fail to occur) when these foods are eaten together.

It is important that when reading any nutrition book you distinguish between general nutrition rules and guidelines and the conditions that must apply to a particular meal.

Food presentation

The West recognizes that the Chinese regard the cutting and shaping of food as important to its appearance. (Also, this art was raised to extremely high aesthetic standards by the Japanese in an art they call "*Mukimono*.")

Paintings can be perceived as an artist's re-creation of a chi pattern, having the attributes of the original chi pattern. This applies to any arrangement of a physical structure, be it a building, painting, or garden. The physical presentation of a meal also contains a chi pattern within that presentation.

Thus, the plate on which a meal is served, the physical layout of the food, the blending of colors, tastes, and aromas — all represent a multidimensional art form that is no less valuable for being transitory.

Presentation is important at every meal. Presentation means more than a pretty plate — it is the creation of a whole "eating" environment. If the diners are uncomfortable they will not benefit as they should. Look at, for example, temperature, ventilation, light, sound, comfort of seating, and space. However, don't look at these things purely from the point of creating a bland environment in which none of them is noticeable — try to create an ambience.

There is a reason restaurants incorporate log fires and artificial fountains in their décor, have appealing views or locations. Generally, when a person is eating out he or she will first look at the restaurant environment and decide if it is "comfortable". Only then will he or she look at menu and price.

Eating

The fourth process involves maintaining or enhancing the quantity of food chi through the food consumption process.

This process dovetails neatly with process three. The food has been carefully selected, prepared, designed, and presented so that it will appeal to all the senses, enhancing its quality. However, now its consumers must play their parts. If you talk through magnificent music, if you give a brilliant picture a cursory glance, you cannot expect to derive much benefit.

As a consumer of a meal you have a similar responsibility to make sure you get the best from it. This should not be a burden, it should be a delight, but, like the creation or appreciation of any art, it requires an ability to focus on what you are doing. Also, the greater the understanding you have of the "art," the greater will be your enjoyment of it and benefit from it.

There are a number of factors involved, including the environment in which you eat and the way in which you consume your food. In general terms, the chi must be settled and the *shen* raised.

Digestion

The fifth process involves maintaining or enhancing the quantity of food chi through the food digestion process.

There are five "areas" of digestion where we can assist the digestive process:

- Mouth: Allow time to eat.
- Stomach: Be aware of food temperature.
- Duodenum: Chew food well, in order to aid saliva production as well as digestion.
- Small intestine: Be aware of emotions when eating, as stress responses inhibit production of digestion-aiding mucous.
- Large intestine: Gentle massaging exercises during the digestive process will aid peristalsis.

A meal is not over when the last mouthful has been ingested. In fact, the time immediately following a meal is critical, for this is when the structural chi is broken down and released within the body.

While everyone appears to agree that vigorous exercise after a meal is not appropriate, there is varying opinion about whether you should rest or partake of mild exercise.

The proponents of rest will often point out that many animals appear to rest after eating. On closer inspection, however, such animals are often carnivores operating on the "feast or famine" principle. That is, a carnivore never really knows where its next meal is coming from and will therefore gorge itself when it does secure a meal. This makes movement uncomfortable for it.

In the case of people, however, it is to be hoped that they will have finished eating when they are about 80 percent replete. In this case, a gentle walk will serve to stimulate the circulatory and energy systems without overexciting them. A stroll in pleasant surroundings can help place the body's energetic systems in a "receptive" state, ideally suited to the digestion of energy as well as of physical food substances. This will aid in proper digestion of food.

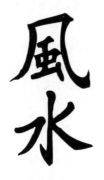

Chapter Seven

Environmental Chi – Feng Shui

WHAT IS FENG SHUI?

FENG SHUI (pronounced "foong shway") is the Chinese chi energy art which deals with the effect of the local environmental chi energy on those living within its area of influence. The Chinese character (or ideogram) for Feng Shui is made up of the symbols for "wind" and "water." To the Chinese, "wind" is often associated with the flow of chi energy; "water" with the storage or accumulation of chi.

The Chinese concept of a universal chi extends back to time immemorial. However, the belief that apparently stimulated the development of Feng Shui as a science was, somewhat paradoxically for a science dealing with life energy, concern about siting of ancestral graves. The Chinese believed that the spirits of their ancestors played a vital role in the lives of their descendants, and the "stronger" a spirit, the more chance it would have to influence its descendants' lives. The best thing the descendants could do to enhance the "strength" of their ancestors' spirits was to ensure their graves were well-situated in respect to the flow of chi.

The Chinese felt that if chi was all-important to the living world then there was no reason for this to be different in the afterlife. This belief eventually became so prevalent that in military campaigns sorties to destroy the graves of the opposing leader's ancestors (to gain a strategic military advantage) became common practice. Re-siting one's own ancestors' graves in a more propitious spot also became a military maneuver. Thus, one of the oldest books containing Feng Shui principles is the *Zhang Shu* (Book of Interment), written during the Jin Dynasty (276–420 AD) by Guo Pu, often regarded as the founder of modern Feng Shui.

Obviously, superstition is a part of such beliefs but virtually all cultures vary only to the degree in which they take an interest in the siting of graves. (It should be stressed that these references to the role of ancestral spirits in the development of Feng Shui are only included for cultural and historical context. The science of Feng Shui is quite independent of whether or not the Chinese speculations on the afterlife were correct.)

Feng Shui continued to gain in popularity. By the Sung Dynasty (960–1126 AD) the role of the specialist Feng Shui expert (*Xiansheng*) existed. While the siting of ancestors' graves was still important, much more attention was now paid to the siting of residences and workplaces, and even to architectural design and interior furnishings. A number of approaches to the practice of Feng Shui developed and there are two major schools of thought today:

- The Kwang Si school: This is the school which is the foundation of this book. Its focus is flows of chi, and how these influence physical surroundings and vice versa.
- The Foh Kien school: This school focuses on the use of what is known as the Feng Shui compass for assessing the quality of chi in a particular locality.

Is Feng Shui a uniquely Chinese discovery or creation? Many cultures have been intuitively aware of the energies that flow throughout the landscape but have not had the unifying concept of chi on which to build a science. Nevertheless, the Chinese were often convinced that some Western builders and architects were not only aware of Feng Shui but were experts in the science, because the buildings that they constructed complied so exactly to Feng Shui requirements. This would suggest that, in some way, people generally are sensitive to the condition of environmental chi, although the level of this sensitivity will vary from person to person.

The Chinese communist government was opposed to such "traditional" beliefs as Feng Shui and tried to suppress its study, particularly during the time of the Cultural Revolution. Feng Shui has, however, continued to spread throughout the world via Chinese communities in many countries.

FENG SHUI AS "ENVIRONMENTAL" SCIENCE

When foreigners first travelled through China they were impressed with the harmony they perceived in the environment around them. Feng Shui was a "green" science long before the word gained its meaning in the modern world of "favoring the environment." However, unlike some contemporary, more extreme, "green" views, Feng Shui did not see humans as interlopers whose very presence damaged the environment. Rather, Feng Shui saw them as an integral part of a complex environmental mechanism that had to be kept in balance.

Indeed, understanding of Feng Shui and sound application of its principles could be used not only to maintain and protect but to improve the natural environment. The very meaning of the term, Feng = Wind and Shui = Water, implies a close connection to the natural environment.

In essence, Feng Shui is about understanding the flow of chi energy in the environment and how to maximize the long-term benefits available from this chi flow. In a contemporary technological and urban society, where the experience and sense of the environment is dulled, anything which promotes an understanding of the connection between people and their environment should be valuable in raising awareness of the need to maintain a proper balance between the two. Global warming and the increasing frequency and severity of natural disasters are signs that such balance is being lost and that people need to improve their stewardship of the planet's resources.

The relationship between humankind and the environment ought to be a mutually beneficial one. However, humans have made so many mistakes with their environment in the past that there seems to be a growing feeling we should be spectators of, not participants in, our environment. This is very dangerous, for it represents the total alienation of people from the environment in which they live.

Environmental mistakes there may have been, but it does not necessarily follow that the answer is to give up and attempt to withdraw from the environment. A walk around some of the great gardens and parks in the world will show that people can interact positively with their environment, to the benefit of both.

Perhaps what must be learned are the principles of environmental interaction. If we look at dam-building, for instance, some environmental catastrophes have occurred. Does this suggest there is something wrong with dam-building, that it necessarily damages the environment? When the common beaver builds its dams the local environment becomes not only richer and more highly speciated but more able to withstand environmental stresses from adverse climatic conditions. Some recent programs in the United States aimed to rebuild beaver populations because doing so not only improves the environment but farmers have found surrounding pasture land increases its carrying capacity and stock becomes healthier.

So, it is not dam-building per se that is wrong, it is how and where the dams are built; it is the principles that are followed. There is no reason why dam-building should be an isolated activity. People may have their cities and roads, but these do not differ in nature from the rookeries built by birds, the nests built by ants and termites or, indeed, the giant coral reefs in which we take such delight. Many animals establish regular paths and tracks; leaf-cutter ants raise crops of fungus. If animals, birds, and coral polyps can enrich the world through carrying out their activities, can't we do the same?

What contemporary human beings have to do is relearn how the environment works — the tao of the environment. Such relearning involves several steps, the first of which requires that we again become aware of the environment, be it natural or artificial. This section of the book explores some exercises to achieve this awareness. Once such awareness is gained, the next step is learning how to obtain benefits from the energy flows in the environment. From this comes the obligation to maintain and enhance the environmental energy flows.

These concepts differ from the chief focus of many Feng Shui books which, when taken out of the full context of Chinese culture, seem almost totally focused on obtaining financial and health benefits for the individual. If Feng Shui — the science of wind and water — is to realize fully the personal and environmental benefits it can create, then it must have its full context; it is not the manipulation of the environment by people for their own benefit but people playing their vital role in the environment (and being benefited as a consequence).

On this basis, many Chinese chi arts are, in fact, Feng Shui arts. Chi gardening and landscape architecture come to mind. These arts aid in the awareness, and the derivation, of benefit from environmental chi. The practice of these arts also leads to the maintenance and improvement of the "energy" environment.

This environment is much bigger than the environment we normally consider. We shall refer to this energy environment as the "chi-scape," since we have no word which is sufficiently inclusive. Chi-scape includes:

External environment
• geophysical forms: mountains, valleys, plains, oceans, rivers, lakes, stars, the sun, the moon, and the planets;
• meteorological conditions: the seasons, rain, storms, the sun, wind, drought, flood, and fire;
• life forms: trees, birds, animals, and people; and
• artifacts: buildings, bridges, and agriculture.

Internal environment
• bodyscape: structure and health of the body and its organs, and energetic and metabolic systems;
• mindscape: willpower, memory, concentration, and intellect; and
• spiritscape: sense of vitality, well-being, emotional balance, moral and ethical conditions, and humanity.

When we consider that all of these factors influence the "chi-scape," we start to appreciate what a complex and sophisticated study Feng Shui is. Here is a quote from a source some 2,500 years old:

Whoever wishes to investigate medicine properly should proceed thus: in the first place, to consider the seasons of the year and what effect each of them produces, for they are not at all alike but differ from themselves in regard to their changes; then the winds, the hot and the cold, especially such as are common to all countries and then such as are peculiar to each locality. We must then consider the qualities of the waters, for as they differ from one another in taste and weight, so do they also differ much in their qualities. In the same manner, when one comes into a city to which he is a stranger, he ought to consider its situation, how it lies as to the winds and the rising of the sun; for its influence is not the same whether it lies to the north or the south, to the rising or the setting sun.

These things one ought to consider most attentively; and concerning the waters which the inhabitants use, whether they be marshy and soft or hard and running from elevated rocky situations, and then if saltish and unfit for cooking; and the ground, whether it be naked and deficient in water or wooded and well-watered and whether it lies in a hollow, confined situation or is elevated and cold.

It might surprise you to know that this is not an ancient Chinese philosopher marrying Feng Shui and other Chinese health arts; it is taken from the Hippocratic writings, by the same Hippocrates whose oath Western doctors still take.

THE BASIC ASSUMPTIONS OF FENG SHUI

It may not immediately be obvious why factors such as the placement of furniture affect our health and well-being. To understand why such decisions are important to Feng Shui we need to understand the assumptions on which Feng Shui rests:

- Chi flow and quality vary with location and physical environment.
- Chi flow and quality in the local environment can affect chi flow and quality within physical structures (including living beings) within that local environment.
- Each state and quality of chi flow has specific effects on physical structures in the local environment. Detection of these effects allows you to make judgments about the state and quality of chi flow in that environment.
- Physical structures can influence the chi flow and quality in the local area. Consequently, it is possible either to change physical structures or to introduce or remove physical structures to or from an area, having specific effects on the state of chi flow and quality in the local environment.

When put this way, there is nothing too esoteric about the science of Feng Shui. If the term chi were replaced with the term "electrical energy," Western science would have no problem with any of these assumptions. The behavior of environmental chi is the same as the behavior of the energies more familiar to the West.

Feng Shui is a little like herbalism, which, when you first look at it, appears to have myriad rules about which herbs are taken in what amounts and which mixtures are for what particular ailments. It is only after long and concentrated study that one is able to distill the logic behind all these remedies.

FENG SHUI THEORY

Feng Shui theory is as simple as the assumptions on which it is built — the physical and energetic local environments affect the state of chi. Therefore, if these environments are examined, some idea of the quantity and quality of chi in the local area can be obtained. Also (within broad limits), by adjusting them, the quantity and quality of local chi can be changed if it is unsatisfactory. Quite likely, when a chi assessment is done of a particular location, it will be found (as with the health of most human beings) that the situation is not ideal. You then have a number of choices:

- **Choosing to tolerate the situation:** Very rarely will we find a perfect chi situation. Like most things, chi adjustment is subject to the law of diminishing returns, that is, the effort to achieve a small adjustment in chi may be out of all proportion to the benefit obtained.

- **Seeking to move to another location:** This would generally apply if the chi condition were having dramatically negative effects on the lives of those in the area and the only chi solutions were very expensive to put into effect.

- **Seeking to modify the flow and quality of chi in the local environment:** In other words, we may effect an "environmental cure." This is really where the science of Feng Shui comes into its own.

The way that an environmental chi "cure" is effected often causes some difficulty in the West. If a particular aspect of the environment is, in medical parlance, simply a "symptom" of an underlying chi problem, how can changing the symptom change the underlying problem?

In actual fact, this happens all the time. In Western medicine, symptoms are often treated. For instance, an excessive temperature may be the result of sunstroke, and artificially lowering the temperature may solve the sunstroke problem altogether. Also, in some ways, matter can be regarded as "captured" or "crystallized" chi. Therefore, by changing the nature of crystallized chi in an area, we are, in fact, changing the balance of the underlying chi in the local environment.

What can surprise Westerners is that the corrective action taken frequently seems quite insignificant and sometimes an attempt to "fool" chi by apparently symbolic acts. For instance, having decided that a slowly flowing river would improve the chi of a particular location, it seems to be cheating to settle for an ornamental pond.

This type of confusion arises from misunderstanding. The fact is, the river and the ornamental pond both reflect chi of the same nature and therefore with the same general effects. Also, whereas the river modifies the chi of the entire landscape through which it flows, the pond has only to modify the chi in the local area — a fraction of the area affected by the river. On a local basis, the chi effect of a pond and river may be similar.

The relationship between chi and the mind must also be considered. The pond may provide a point of focus for the mind and spirit that allows either for a considerable effect on the actual chi of the area, or on the ability of the body to prevent the environmental chi problems from interacting with it.

For instance, when a Chinese person creates a painting, he or she may regard it as capturing the chi in the environment the painting represents. Thus, the picture itself can exert (on a smaller scale) the same sort of influences on local chi flow as the environmental aspects it represents (as we shall see in the section on environmental cures below).

Feng Shui "si jian"

How do we assess the condition and quality of environmental chi? We look at the health and vitality of a place as we would the health and vitality of a person.

If a Chinese doctor were conducting an examination, he or she would perform the *si jian* — four examinations:

- looking;
- listening;
- questioning; and
- touching.

It is appropriate to take the same approach with the environment, and perform a Feng Shui *si jian* in order to assess the state of chi in a particular location.

Let us see if the four examinations performed by a doctor have any parallels with what can be done to assess energy conditions and quality in a location.

Looking

A doctor looks at a person's color, physical appearance generally, and at how he or she moves. These are appropriate Feng Shui concerns.

- Color/light: Does the location get too much or too little direct sunlight? Do the rooms allow in too little or too much natural light? How would one describe the rooms and the total effect of their lighting and color schemes — harsh, bright and cheerful, or gloomy and depressing?

- Physical appearance: What impression do you get of the location, building, and furnishings — heavy or light, strong or flimsy, stable or impermanent?

- Movement: What is the nature of the movement of air, water, people, and transportation in the area — is it animated or is the place lifeless?

Listening

A doctor focuses on a person's voice (that is, the volume and rate of speech) and the sound of his or her heart and breathing. The doctor would also use his or her sense of smell. Again, this is applicable to a Feng Shui examination.

- Sounds: Are any sounds you hear pleasant or disturbing in their nature or volume? What do they indicate about the nature of the location? Do you perceive the presence of pleasant activities and life forms or disagreeable ones?

- Smell: Pay particular attention to smell. Are any odors you notice fresh, pleasant, and stimulating, or are they unpleasant and indicative of problems?

Questioning

A doctor asks questions to find out what cannot be seen or heard by examination but which may give insights into the person's condition, for example, questions about diet, activities, or traumatic events the person may have experienced. Again, there are analogous questions in respect to a Feng Shui examination:

- Climate: Is the area subject to a lot of wind, storms, and/or rain? Are its winters and summers harsh?
- Uses: Have the land or buildings been put to particular agricultural and/or industrial uses?
- Atmosphere: Is the area particularly prone to sickness? Does it have a good "reputation?" What sort of events have happened there?

Touching

His or her sense of touch can tell a doctor a great deal about the person being examined. It can also be useful in a Feng Shui examination. If a place feels either cold and damp or hot and dry, the condition of chi may be poor. Such conditions should be avoided, modified, or compensated for.

In most cases there will be a whole range of good and bad indications, and you will have to form an overall assessment of the chi flow and quality.

"Eight conditions" Feng Shui cures method

Chi "cures" can be categorized as yin/yang adjustments. The most productive approach for the non-expert in Feng Shui would be to know the "conditions" in which an excess or deficiency of environmental chi could be identified, as well as some ways of correcting any such excesses or deficiencies.

We will now look at the "eight conditions cures approach." This is closely connected to the Feng Shui *si jian* environmental chi examination, and basically allows chi problems to be identified on the basis of eight particular conditions. That is, an excess or deficiency of, and high or low quality in the:

- light energy condition;
- sound energy condition;
- thermal energy condition;
- moisture energy condition;
- bio-energy condition;
- aroma energy condition;
- moving energy condition; and the
- crystallized energy condition.

We will now look briefly at the type and nature of chi "cures" available for each of these conditions.

Light energy condition
Excess condition cures are as follows:
*   decreasing the number of windows and light entrances, either physically or effectively (by use of shades, drapes, blinds);
*   tinting, frosting, or staining windows;
*   using light-absorbent furniture and fittings;
*   using subdued colors; and
*   planting shade trees and erecting shade screens.

Deficiency condition cures are as follows:
*   increasing window size;
*   having brighter, glossier colors on walls, ceilings, floors, and furnishings;
*   using colorful pictures, especially those depicting brightly lit landscapes;
*   increasing internal lighting; and
*   using mirrors and crystals to draw in light energy.

Quality-raising cures are as follows:
*   using crystals;
*   filtering light through trees;
*   using water reflections; and
*   changing the light-mix so there is more natural, rather than artificial, light.

Sound energy condition
Excess condition cures are as follows:
*   installing insulation, either natural (through vegetation barriers) or structural; and
*   placing a source of pleasant sound before a source of excess noise. Fountains and waterfalls can be effective, as can music.

Deficiency condition cures are as follows:
*   using vegetation to generate wind sounds;
*   hanging wind chimes;
*   encouraging birds and pleasant-sounding insects (bees);

- introducing water sounds through fountains and artificial waterfalls; and
- playing music.

Quality-raising cures are as follows:
- all deficiency condition cures also increase sound quality.

Thermal energy condition (hot/cold)

Excess condition cures are as follows:
- ensuring there is sufficient shade;
- installing insulation;
- using cool colors;
- putting in fountains and pools;
- using "cool" materials such as rock and stone; and
- installing fans and cooling devices.

Deficiency condition cures are as follows:
- using warm colors;
- installing insulation;
- installing internal heating; and
- creating sun-traps.

Quality-raising cures are as follows:
- changing the heating mix so there is more natural heating from sun and insulation than there is from combustion and electrical devices.

Moisture energy condition

Excess condition cures are as follows:
- increasing the amount of low-growing vegetation with high water requirements. Avoiding trees with dense foliage cover;
- improving drainage;
- increasing air flow; and
- using dehumidifiers and, where appropriate, heating.

Deficiency condition cures are as follows:
- externally — planting large shade trees;
- internally — having house plants; and
- putting in waterfalls and fountains.

Quality-raising cures are as follows:
- ensuring moisture comes from vegetation rather than

ground soil; and
- ensuring moisture comes from moving, rather than still, water.

Bio-energy condition

Excess condition cures are as follows (this generally only results from too many people and too much activity in the local area):
- planting vegetation barriers; and
- erecting walls and fences.

Deficiency condition cures are as follows:
- increasing the amount of internal and external vegetation;
- keeping pets;
- keeping fish — indoors and out; and
- attracting birds through the use of appropriate feeders and vegetation.

Quality-raising cures are as follows:
- ensuring health and vitality of plants and animals.

Aroma energy condition

Excess condition cures are as follows:
- eliminating the source of the aroma;
- increasing ventilation, if the aroma is in a building;
- masking the aroma with aromatic plants;
- using incense; and
- using chemical absorbents.

Deficiency condition cures are as follows:
- planting aromatic plants, herbs, and trees;
- using aromatic materials, such as timber, in buildings and furnishings; and
- using incense and scents.

Quality-raising cures are as follows:
- eliminating bad aromas at their source rather than masking them; and
- making sure aromas come from natural, rather than unnatural, sources.

Moving energy condition

Excess condition cures are as follows:
- putting in windbreaks, through planting vegetation or

building fences and walls. (Windbreaks are effective against all types of moving chi.)

Deficiency condition cures are as follows:

- putting in waterfalls or fountains, hanging mobiles or pendulum clocks;
- planting vegetation that moves in light breezes; and
- installing fans, especially large ceiling fans.

Quality-raising cures are as follows:

- ensuring movement is from natural, rather than unnatural, sources; and
- ensuring movement has depth and momentum, rather than high speed and irregularity. (Irregularity relates to the power of the movement rather than the direction; mobiles or wind-moved trees would not move in a regular direction.)

Crystallized energy condition

Excess condition cures are as follows:

- where physical structures are too massive, supplementing them with smaller structures and living things; and
- using any of the cures that involve movement.

Deficiency condition cures are as follows:

- putting in place large stones and rocks and "massive" furniture — anything which anchors chi; and
- internally, putting in pictures of mountain scenes, statues, and heavy sculptures.

Quality-raising cures are as follows:

- focusing on natural "cures."

Summary

From the above we derive the following conclusions:

- The flow of environmental chi energy varies from place to place.
- In some places chi energy will flow in a manner which enhances the health and well-being of the individual and the environment.
- In other places the environmental chi flow will be too

weak or too strong and this will have an adverse effect on the health and well-being of the individual environment.

People have a responsibility to take actions which maintain and improve the local chi environment.

- The Feng Shui *si jian* may be used to determine the local flow and quality of chi.
- The eight conditions cures method may be used to create the most favorable chi environment possible.

CHI AND LANDSCAPES

As previously mentioned, the nature of the landforms in the local area can be seen both to indicate the nature of the local chi energy and to modify the chi energy passing through the area.

Landforms are created through tectonic forces existing within the earth's crust. These landforms are then modified by the forces of erosion, that is, by wind and water. Landscape can therefore be seen as an indication of the collision of various energies; chi is the primal energy which moves and motivates these other energies. We can thus look at landscape to give us a picture of the underlying energy movements and, from this, deduce their likely effect on the chi of the area and the people who dwell within it.

To determine the effect of a landform on the Feng Shui of an object, you must first determine the relationship of that object to the landform. The significance of the positional relationship can be understood by using the following analogy. Place a metal object in the field of a magnet. If you place the object above the magnet, the apparent weight of the object is increased. If you place it below the magnet, its apparent weight is decreased. In any direction, the magnet and object will tend to move towards each other but the direction of movement will depend on the relative positions. In the same way, the chi effect of a landform will vary, depending on the location of the landform.

As a general rule, the closer an object is to a landform, the greater the influence on the object's chi. (No allowance is made for vertical variations. Thus, for instance, with a forty-storey skyscraper, the influence of a landform on the tenth storey and the twentieth storey is not to be deemed different, unless the distances are significant. This would be consistent with the chi fields generated by landforms having a polar nature.)

SITUATING BUILDINGS IN RELATION
TO CHI FLOWS

When Feng Shui was first practiced, one of the main concerns of its followers was the situation of buildings in respect to natural chi flows. These chi flows were seen in the flow of water in a river, in the direction of the prevailing wind, and in a building's position in respect to the energy from the sun.

It was generally considered that when these pathways were directed at a building, unfortunate consequences could follow if the flow of chi became too strong. In fact, this chi was often referred to as "evil" — *sha chi*.

This is obviously common sense. If you build a house in line with the flow of a river, that is, facing the direction of the river on the outer side of a curve in the river, you are building in an area that is most prone to flood and erosion, because it is here that the force of the river is directed.

Similarly, building on the side of a hill facing prevailing winds, or building so that a house faces the full force of the sun in a hot climate, has ill effects on the dwelling and its inhabitants. The Feng Shui of an area would also be judged according to its geology — houses would be situated to avoid fault lines and dry watercourses. Again, this plainly makes sense.

It is interesting, however, that people often choose to build cities in areas where high energy conditions sometimes exist. Thus, for instance, cities such as San Francisco and Los Angeles are situated next to fault lines, which periodically have devastating consequences. (One cannot blame this on ignorant Western practices because San Francisco has the largest Chinese population in the United States!) It would seem that, in the absence of earthquakes, the normal energy conditions of these cities is great enough to make them productive and beneficial places. A useful analogy is the River Nile, where the problems caused by the annual floods have been more than offset by the value of the silt deposited on the agricultural land.

However, these days the significant chi flows in the local environment are likely to be generated by artificial structures such as roads and railways. As discussed earlier, chi is very much like water in that its progress is slowed by bends and obstructions. Straight roads therefore speed the flow of chi, but many roads end in "T-shape" intersections. This directs chi, at high speed, into the area opposite the stem of the "T" so these roads are generally not regarded as good ones in which to

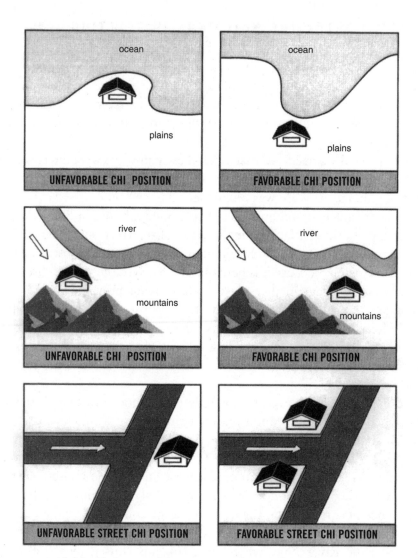

live, particularly if the road becomes wider and/or busier.

The nature of the local environment determines the nature of the chi energy that reaches a dwelling, but the nature of the building determines the amount of the energy which enters inside. Consider, for instance, a building facing a major T-intersection. If that dwelling has no fence, a flat lawn without trees and bushes, and a large floor-to-ceiling picture window (without blinds or curtains) that faces directly down the road, then the negative influence of the *sha chi* will be much higher than if there is a brick wall, backed with trees, creating a courtyard effect around the window to the house. Alternatively, the window can have thickened glass (lead-lighting would be excellent), drapes can be hung, and pot plants can be placed just inside the window.

It is the total effect that is important, not an individual feature. For instance, the effect of facing a T-intersection at the bottom of a hill is very different to being at the top of a hill. In fact, if traffic volume is low and the hill is steep, the location at the bottom could, quite possibly, reflect a deficiency of energy.

The final factor is what happens to the chi energy once it is in a dwelling. How is it circulated and influenced? This is when interior design and furnishings become important.

BUILDING AND LANDFORM SHAPE IN RESPECT TO THE FIVE ENERGIES

The role of the five element theory with regard to Feng Shui will not be entered into here, in so far as it is best left to the trained practitioner. However, the following is included to demonstrate the part that the theory plays in the type of chi energy inspired by building and landform shapes.

Wood

Columnar mountains and hills (such as those found around Guilin); buildings such as skyscrapers and towers, and chimneys; rectangular structures standing on their shorter side. Wood symbolizes energy that expands in all directions, and many corporate headquarters are found in buildings of this nature. On the other hand, such structures should not contain residences.

The dragon is a figure of stability. It symbolizes wisdom.

Fire

Upward-moving energy; sharp-peaked mountains; pyramidal and cone-shaped buildings, such as those with spires, used by many religions to draw energy in. (The actual place of worship or meditation is rarely spire-shaped internally.)

Associated with the bird and the obvious image of flight. The bird is often thought of as the phoenix, the bird that never dies (or is constantly reborn).

Earth

Plains, prairies, flat depressions; low, flat-topped buildings as in factory sheds; cube-type shapes. Energy is neither expansive nor contractive; rather, it moves around its own axis. Suburban landscapes can be regarded as earth-like. Many residential dwellings have this format.

Earth is the snake. It directs, yet is protected by, the other four creatures.

Metal

Rounded hills; houses with domes; aircraft hangar-shaped buildings (metal energy gathers internally, and is often associated with storage places); geodesic domes. Many governmental buildings have large domes.

The tiger is associated with strength. (Interestingly, the tiger is also associated with repressed violence.)

Water

Lakes, rivers, ponds; irregular buildings, as long as they are not too angular. Many castles and fortifications followed this pattern, often emphasized by crenellated walls and round towers. Many universities consisted of buildings to which, because of their complexity, it was difficult to ascribe a shape. Schools often have similar complicated, interlocked structures. Water energy descends for points of maximum concentration.

The tortoise symbolizes security. It is a place of gathering, from whence the cycle will start all over again.

FENG SHUI EXERCISE

It has previously been explained that Feng Shui is the science of understanding environmental chi and using this understanding to maximize both the state of "health" of one's personal chi and the local environmental chi.

Exercise is one of life's most important activities and, like all other activities, is carried out in, and thus is interactive with, the environment. The only choice you have is whether when you exercise you do so conscious of this connection. In this sense, all exercises could be described as, to some degree, Feng Shui exercise. However, the maximum effect of Feng Shui exercises will be achieved when the practitioner seeks to:

- select carefully the most suitable chi environment in which to perform the exercise;
- modify the chi environment (as far as is possible) when it is not ideal;
- change the exercises (in order to reduce any adverse effect on the practitioners) where the chi environment cannot be modified sufficiently; and
- perform the exercises in a manner which leaves the local chi environment improved.

Let us look at each of these.

Selecting the environment

It is fascinating that, in general, people almost instinctively seek out locations with good environmental chi in which to perform their exercises. Thus (even though the exercise may not require much space), during the daytime people will generally choose to exercise out of doors if the weather conditions are not extreme. When they exercise outdoors they are far more likely to choose a park, a riverside, or an ocean frontage. This is particularly so in the case of Chinese exercises (wherever in the world they are performed).

The Feng Shui *si jian* technique previously referred to is one of the most effective ways of assessing the local environmental chi to determine whether it is a good place to exercise. However, there are a number of other factors that should be taken into account when selecting an exercise or an exercise location from an environmental chi perspective:

- It is not only the current condition of the environmental chi but how it is changing which is important. Consider the season and the time of day when you are selecting an exercise for a particular location (or a location for a particular exercise).
- Do not forget to take into account your own energy or chi condition. What is your age? What is your condition of health (physically, mentally, emotionally, and spiritually)? For instance, if your energy needs a lift, exercising beside a strongly flowing waterfall may be appropriate. If you are overstressed or hyperactive,

exercising in a quiet park or by a lake would be better.
That is, if you are suffering yin energy conditions seek
out yang energy locations and vice versa.

All this does not mean that you have to perform a scientific
examination of the location every time you want to exercise. Rather, try
to develop an awareness of energy flow and movement around you. To
some extent you have to learn to trust your intuition; what feels right,
probably is right. Without any theory or special knowledge people seek
out parks and riversides where they can perform their Tai Chi in the
early morning or early evening, and they tend to exercise more in spring
and autumn than they do in the depths of winter or at the height of
summer. All of this makes eminent sense in terms of chi principles.

A few simple guidelines:

- Areas with large trees and healthy plant growth are
  generally indicative of good chi, so the selection of a
  park is fairly natural. Slow, meandering rivers are also
  associated with good chi.
- Waterfalls, cascades, and white-water areas all raise the
  energy level, but be careful to ensure that the overall
  energy level is not too high.
- Avoid extremes of heat and cold, dryness and moisture,
  and keep out of the wind.

Wind, in particular, has the ability to disrupt chi seriously. (You will
often see animals and children display erratic behavior in windy
conditions.) Wind also has an effect on the body's *wei chi*, leaving you
vulnerable to infection, and is often associated with headaches.

Modifying the environment

We cannot always exercise in a park or on a riverbank; often we must
exercise inside buildings. If our Feng Shui *si jian* indicates chi problems,
we may be able to take corrective actions best indicated by the eight
conditions cures method previously described.

As far as indoor exercise areas are concerned, pay special attention
to the:

- Light energy condition: Make use of whatever natural
  light is available, and light should be low if it is
  artificially-based; colorful pictures/posters, flowers, and
  other decorations can make a substantial difference.

- Thermal energy condition: Ensure heating or cooling systems are properly operational, although, if possible, avoid the use of such artificial systems — use clothing and fans to achieve the desired results.
- Moving energy condition: This is likely to be too low. Open windows and doors where possible; add fans and pictures involving movement.
- Bio-energy condition: This is likely to be low. Use plants and floral displays.
- Sound energy condition: Likely to be deadened, with only artificial and disruptive sounds. Play music or nature sounds in the background.

(Do not exercise outdoors in "excessive" heat, cold, damp, dryness, or wind. If you must do so, keep the time to a minimum and wear suitable protective clothing.)

Changing the exercises

For instance, in cold environments increase warm-ups, use moving meditation, and reduce still meditation. In hot environments decrease exercise necessitating high physical exertion and increase meditation. In damp and windy conditions, exercise is best avoided.

Performing the exercises

Naturally, any activity which physically damages the environment will leave the chi environment damaged. While the environment can repair itself, every effort should be made to ensure that the location chosen is appropriate for the type of exercise and that the environment is not subject to excessive stress.

LEVEL OF FENG SHUI SKILLS REQUIRED TO IMPROVE HEALTH AND WELL-BEING

Having considered how to diagnose and prescribe cures for environmental chi problems, it is perhaps appropriate to consider whether this is a job for the "non-expert."

Feng Shui as a science is not inherently difficult to understand and can be predicted from the Feng Shui assumptions about the behavior of chi. Nevertheless, just as we would expect a person (be he or she educated in Chinese or Western medicine) to be very well-trained before trying to deal with serious or subtle health conditions, so are there "experts" in Feng Shui who deal with the more serious or subtle problems that develop with energy flows and energy balance.

However, to continue the analogy, just as ordinary individuals can handle simple health problems such as colds, stomach disorders and minor cuts and bruises through application of some simple rules and knowledge, so, too, can ordinary individuals use basic Feng Shui knowledge and principles to improve their lives.

Just as health practitioners recognize that individuals must take responsibility for their own health (rather than see the doctor after the damage has been done), it is important that the individual take responsibility for the local chi environment. If individuals become attuned to their environment and are able to recognize what damages it and what enhances it, and take the appropriate action, much will have been gained.

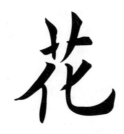

Chapter Eight

The Lotus

INTRODUCTION

THE LOTUS RELAXATION AND BODY TONING EXERCISE is a Tai Chi Qigong, that is, a sequence of movements to exercise the body and mind which is combined with deep diaphragmatic breathing. It follows Tai Chi principles except that it involves full extension of the limbs in stretching movements.

The Lotus is a particularly beneficial form of Tai Chi Qigong, and especially useful for children, because it is easy to learn and significant benefits may be gained for little effort. Using mental imagery makes it easy to remember the sequences and, at the same time, creates a relaxed and positive mood.

HISTORY

Throughout China thousands seek out their favorite spots in which to perform their early morning exercise. As you walk through the streets and parks you can see hundreds of different exercises being practiced — Tai Chi, Pa Kua, Hsing-I, Tao Yin, Qigong — to name but a few. Some of these exercise sets have been handed down within families for centuries; only the quality of the performance distinguishes the amateur from the Grandmaster.

Early one morning when I was out practicing, I saw an old man performing a set of postures I had not seen before. Day after day I watched the old master going through the same movements. Finally, I introduced myself to him and asked about the origins of this exercise art.

Although many in China guard their art jealously (which has actually resulted in much valuable knowledge being lost), the old master was happy not only to discuss his art, but to teach it to me. Over time I researched and worked on these movements and evolved them into a continuous Qigong (Chi Kung) form, which I called the Lotus.

Jou Tsung Hwa in *The Tao of Tai Chi Chuan —Way to Rejuvenation* refers to an exercise set containing fourteen postures, which he describes only as a Tai Chi Qigong. The Lotus movements are very similar to eleven of these postures (the exceptions being the loss of the "Press against the Wind" movement and the addition of a number of movements where only the head is turned). However, the movements have no names and so there is no incorporation of mental imagery. The existence of these moves, however, does suggest that:

- the exercise set which was the origin of the Lotus was not simply one belonging to a family, but had considerable tradition behind it;
- the fact that the ordering of the moves is the same (even though in Jou's rendition there is no particular reason why one posture should follow another) indicates the sequence has an underlying importance.

Jou is quite laudatory about the benefits of the set of Tai Chi Qigong containing fourteen postures, saying that by practicing it the student of Tai Chi Chuan is far more likely to master the art. This is in part because the Tai Chi Qigong helps him or her build up inner energy.

What better introduction could there be to the Lotus!

BENEFITS

As a Tai Chi Qigong exercise the Lotus is more than an exercise for muscles and tendons; it is an internal art which has the capacity to benefit all of the body and mind functions. The reference to "Tai Chi" tells us that this is an exercise involving the balancing and bringing into harmony of the elementary forces of yin and yang, and the reference to "Qigong" tells us that the exercise involves chi (vital energy).

The benefits of the Lotus can be summarized as follows:

- **Relaxation and stress reduction:** The "stretch and

release" technique used in the Lotus aids in releasing tensions that have built up in muscle tissue. The deep diaphragmatic breathing also helps to relax the body, normalizing blood pressure. Finally, the use of imagery relaxes the mind.

- **Cardiovascular stimulation:** While there are no stepping patterns in the Lotus, the sequence of movements involves continually raising and lowering the body by bending the knees. This ensures the leg muscles alternately tense and relax. Since venous blood vessels thread through the leg musculature, the venous blood returns to the torso by the action of the muscles rather than the heart doing all the work. (For a more detailed analysis of exercise and the venous blood return system, refer to Senior Master Gary Khor, *Tai Chi Qigong — For Stress Control and Relaxation,* Chapter 4.) The cardiovascular load imposed by this exercise is small enough to be safe but big enough to promote improvement in the capacity of the cardiovascular system to cope with stress imposed by sudden physical demands.

- **Breathing:** The exercise promotes the use of diaphragmatic breathing. This makes the physical lung capacity greater, increasing the amount of oxygen sent into the bloodstream with each breath. It also helps to ensure that carbon dioxide and other toxins are more fully expelled from the lower parts of the lung, where they may otherwise accumulate. Generally, the use of the diaphragm to breathe, and the increase in the contraction and expansion of the lungs, has a massaging effect on the internal organs that improves their supply of blood, getting more oxygen to them and effectively removing waste products faster. (For a more detailed analysis of how diaphragmatic breathing benefits the body, refer to *Tai Chi Qigong — For Stress Control and Relaxation,* Chapter 2.)

- **Posture:** the exercise encourages good posture, which helps protect the spine and neck, and may assist in avoiding or managing backache and posturally related headaches.

- **The traditional Chinese health perspective:** the exercise promotes the circulation of chi within the body. The breathing increases the air chi absorbed; the stretching promotes increased flow of chi within the meridians, which promotes the health of the internal organs; the imagery helps to raise and refine the *shen* (emotional balance and feeling of well-being); and the physical movements help tone the body, increasing *li* (strength).

LEARNING THE LOTUS

The Lotus is quite easy to learn, with many people having done so simply by following the movements of others. Those who are encountering the Lotus for the first time, or who are not yet proficient in the exercise, are recommended to approach it as follows:

- Run through the movement instructions. At this stage do not worry about the breathing (just breathe naturally), the stretching, or the "important points." Just concentrate on getting a general idea of the movements and learning the associated imagery. This will make the sequence easier to master.
- When you can perform the full sequence of movements, add the breathing pattern. When you have mastered the breathing pattern, focus on the "important points."
- Finally, work on developing the stretching movements in the set.

Lotus can be used as a stand-alone health exercise system for relaxation and general health improvement, or it can be used in conjunction with other exercise systems as a warming-up or cooling-down routine.

If you are using the Lotus as a stand-alone exercise it is recommended that you perform the sequence several times, so as to get twenty minutes of continuous exercise; this will result in greater cardiovascular benefit. Also, greater stimulation of the endocrine system brings deeper relaxation.

For those who have limited mobility and cannot stand (or find it difficult to), the exercise can be performed from a seated position, as long as there is sufficient space to move the arms freely. The spine should be straight and a "mental intention" to rise or fall should replace the bending and straightening of the legs.

PRINCIPLES

Movement

All movements should be slow, interconnected, and unforced. Use the Tai Chi principle of "reeling silk," that is, imagine you are pulling a strand of silk from a silkworm's cocoon.

Breathing

Use diaphragmatic breathing throughout:

- Breathe in and out through the nose. Keep lips closed, with teeth slightly apart so that the jaw is relaxed.
- Direct the breath down to the *tan tien* and feel the abdomen, not the chest, expand when you breathe in. Mentally follow the breath down to the *chi hai* point (three finger-widths below the navel); the mind acts as an observer, not a director. At no point should the breath be held or forced, since this will only increase tension.

It may help to visualize the breath as a stream of air, flowing on the breath in from the nose, down the throat, along the front centerline of the body to the *chi hai* point and, on the breath out, from the *chi hai* point to the spine, up the back, to the top of the head, then down to the nose and out.

Another technique is to "listen" to the breath, and let it become quieter, softer, and smoother. In Chinese parlance, to listen means to use all the senses of the body, not just the hearing. So, be aware of how the breath feels as it moves through the nose and throat and into and out of the lungs.

A breathing pattern is provided for each Lotus movement. However, the Lotus is also an excellent vehicle for practicing many Qigong breathing techniques. (For a more detailed discussion of diaphragmatic breathing, refer to *Tai Chi Qigong – For Stress Control and Relaxation*, Chapter 2.)

Posture

In all moves except "Press the Earth" use the principle of "suspended headtop," where the spine is kept perpendicular, the head is held as though lifted from the center of its crown, and the coccyx is tucked under. The shoulders are relaxed.

Stretching

Unlike Tai Chi, the Lotus uses stretches; but these should not be forced or put pressure on joints. To stretch more, repeat the sequence three or more times, gradually increasing the amount of stretching each time.

The stretches are an important part of the Lotus and descriptions are given in the movement instructions. The arms, legs, and torso are stretched, with the leg stretch occurring when the legs are straightened. The stretch is designed for the muscles not the knee joints, so try to keep the knees slightly off-lock when you straighten the legs.

The stretching should be as much in the mind as in the body, with use of the "mental intention" to stretch and reach. This is important because there are two sets of muscles in the body, flexors and extensors. The flexors move the limbs back in towards the body and the extensors move the limbs out into the stretched position. If you mentally try to "pull back" an extension of the limbs at the same time as you are stretching, it is possible to activate both these sets of muscles at once, that is, the muscles work against each other. This gives them the sort of workout that they would normally only have during the type of stretch that could put the joints at risk. It takes a little bit of practice, but this is a safer and healthier way of stretching. Use of mind intention in this way also encourages chi flow.

Holistic approach

The Lotus exercises all aspects of the body and mind:
- *shen* (emotion/spirit), through use of mental imagery;
- *yi* (willpower/intellect), through concentration on the form and principles of the movement;
- *li* (physical systems of the body — muscles, tendons, ligaments), through full use of stretches and posture; and
- *chi* (vital energy), through breathing and mental direction of the movements.

Take your time over preparation, do not rush to embark on the Lotus movements themselves. Remember: "Stillness comes before motion."

PREPARATION

This movement aligns the body posture, ensuring that it is upright but relaxed. It also calms the breathing so that it is centered, and focuses the mind, so that you are concentrated and prepared.

Movement breakdown

Movements

1. Commence in a standing position with feet side by side and arms hanging loosely.
2. Lower the body by bending the knees slightly. Slowly raise left knee just high enough for the foot to clear the floor, and step a little less than a shoulder-width to the left. Weight is now centered equally between both feet.

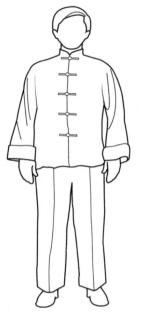

Breathing

Breathe out as you lower the body.

Breathe in as you raise the body, stepping left.

Breathe out as you lower the body after stepping left.

Mental imagery

Preparation requires no specific mental imagery.

Important points

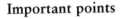

- Feet are parallel.
- Knees are off-lock.
- Shoulders are relaxed.
- Spine is straight, with the head lifted through the *bai hui* point (the center of the crown of the head).
- Stepping wider than a shoulder-width stance can make balancing difficult in the gentle upward stretches.

WAVING HANDS

This movement stretches the spine, tones the muscles, releases muscular tensions, and improves blood circulation. It also increases energy levels and activates the cerebral functions, as well as being calming emotionally. It follows on from Preparation.

Movement breakdown

Movements

1. Draw your mental focus inwards.
2. To commence, arms are relaxed with palms facing backwards.
3. Slowly sweep arms forwards and upwards until hands are extended at shoulder height with fingertips pointing forwards and palms facing downwards. Keep shoulders relaxed.
4. Lower the body by bending the knees as far as is comfortable. At the same time relax the stretch by slowly lowering the elbows, then gently push hands downwards until they are about waist height.

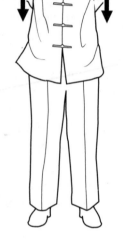

Breathing

Breathe in as you raise the hands.
Breathe out as you lower the body and then lower the hands.

Mental imagery

Before you commence the movements, perform the following visualization (with eyes open or closed, and breathing deeply and naturally):

Imagine that it is very early in the morning and you are in the country, standing on a grassy hilltop. It is that magical moment just before dawn when you get a sense of quietness and stillness, and you are looking out towards the horizon. It is very peaceful.

As you mentally see the sun rise, slowly open your eyes, retaining your visualization of the rising sun. Follow the rising sun with your hands, almost as though they are drawing the sun up.

As you bring your hands down, visualize the country scene around you being illuminated by the sun's light: it is one of rolling green hills and, at your feet, a gentle, meandering stream.

Important points

- Keep the body vertical.
- Do not over-stretch.
- Keep shoulders relaxed.
- Do not curl fingers.

TURTLE TREADS WATER

This movement increases cardiovascular fitness, the diaphragmatic breathing improving lung capacity. It also expands your mental horizons, bringing you feelings of serenity. It follows on from Waving Hands.

Movement breakdown

Movements

1. The hands are hanging down at the sides. Roll palms to face upwards, fingertips pointing towards the front.
2. Draw both hands backwards into the waist, then sweep them outwards and upwards, bringing them to shoulder height. Arms are outstretched, palms face downwards, and fingertips point outwards to each side.
3. Continue arc of the hands until arms face directly forwards, fingertips pointing forwards, palms facing downwards.
4. Continue movement of the hands by bending arms inward at elbows and crossing forearms over each other at shoulder height, palms facing downwards. Fingertips of the right arm point left and fingertips of the left arm point right.
5. Raise the body by straightening the legs. At the same time angle palms outwards and sweep arms outwards, until they are extended to the sides at shoulder height. Arms are fully stretched, with fingertips pointing outwards to the sides and palms angled to the rear. (This movement has a similar feel to the breast stroke in swimming.)

Breathing

Breathe in as you bring the hands in front of the body.
Breathe out as you raise the body and bring the hands to the sides.

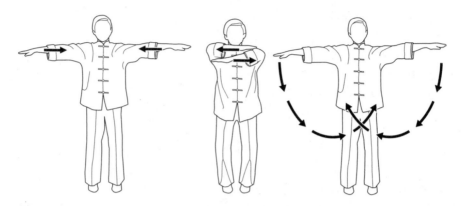

Mental imagery

Imagine you are a turtle in a stream. Feel the cool invigoration of the water; as you sweep your hands forwards in the swimming motion, feel the water on your palms as you push it away from you.

Important points

- In this exercise particularly, keep shoulders relaxed.
- Keep knees bent until commencing the swimming motion.

SNOW RABBIT DIGS THE EARTH

This movement exercises the shoulders and elbows, strengthens the abdominal muscles, and straightens the spine. It is also beneficial to the digestive system. It follows on from Turtle Treads Water.

Movement breakdown
Movements

1. Lower the body by relaxing the knees. At the same time arc arms downwards and forwards. Arms cross at wrists in front of the centerline of the body about navel height, palms angled towards the body, fingertips pointing slightly outwards at an angle with the ground.
2. Lift the crossed hands in front of the body until elbows are about chest height. Keeping elbows down, continue raising the crossed hands until they are face height, palms facing forwards, fingertips pointing upwards.

3. Keeping wrists crossed, roll hands forward in a downward arc until palms come to face the body.
4. Continue arcing movement, drawing hands up the center of the body. As the backs of the hands face forwards, separate hands so that arms extend in front at shoulder height, a shoulder-width apart, palms facing up and fingertips pointing to the front. Feel the stretch.
5. Raise the body by straightening the legs. At the same time relax the stretch, arcing hands downwards until they are slightly to the rear of the body, palms facing forwards and fingertips downwards.

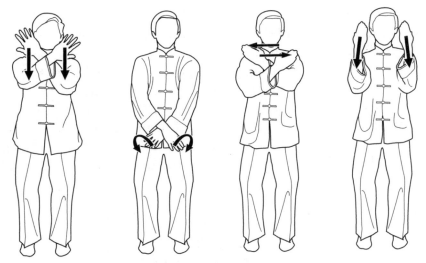

Breathing
Breathe in as you bring the hands up in front of the body.
Breathe out as you draw the hands down.
Breathe in as you roll the hands forward.
Breathe out as you separate the hands and draw them down.

Mental imagery
Imagine you are a rabbit, foraging on the banks of a stream in the early morning. As your hands roll forwards, feel yourself scooping through soft, moist earth.

Important points

- It is most important to keep shoulders relaxed throughout. If this is difficult, lower elbows.

FAIR MAIDEN SCOOPS WATER

This movement exercises the arms and chest and improves the breathing and lung capacity. Mentally, it should expand your awareness and outlook. It follows on from Snow Rabbit Digs the Earth.

Movement breakdown
Movements

1. Lower the body by bending the knees slightly. At the same time "cup" palms, as though trying to hold as much water as possible in them. Take hands forwards and upwards to shoulder height, fingertips pointing forwards, palms facing upwards.
2. Raise the body by straightening the legs. At the same time roll wrists so that fingertips face each other, and separate fingers, as though allowing water to run through them. Then arc hands out to shoulder height, fingertips pointing to each side, palms facing up. Feel the stretch.

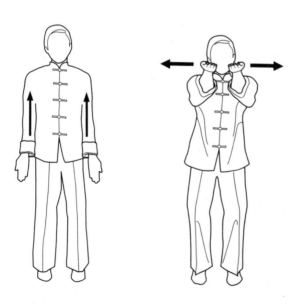

Breathing
Breathe in as you raise the hands in front of the body.
Breathe out as you stretch the arms out to the sides.

Mental imagery
Imagine yourself coming down to a stream. Plunge your hands into the water, scooping it up in your palms and then allowing it to run through your fingers as you sweep your arms out to the sides. Focus on the cooling, refreshing feel of the water in your palms and the sensation it gives as it runs through your fingers.

Important points

* Keep shoulders relaxed.

RAINDROPS FALL ON LOTUS

This movement exercises the shoulders and arms, and stretches and relaxes the spine. It also stimulates the flow of energy, and focuses and centers concentration. It follows on from Fair Maiden Scoops Water.

Movement breakdown
Movements
1. Arc hands upwards so that arms are raised above the head, fingertips pointing to the sky and palms facing each other, shoulder-width apart. Feel the stretch.
2. Curl fingers into the palms to form cotton fists (that is, pretend you are enfolding a small bird's egg in each hand; there should be no pressure or tension in the fists).
3. Lower the body by bending the knees slightly. At the same time draw elbows down until fists are about ear height or lower. Feel the downward stretch in the shoulder.

Breathing
Breathe in as you raise the hands up over the head.
Breathe out as you lower the body and draw the elbows down.

Mental imagery
Imagine clouds gathering overhead as your arms sweep upwards, and a gentle rain falling as you bring your fists down and bend your knees.

Important points

- Keep shoulders relaxed.
- Do not tense hands or wrists when forming fists.

LOTUS FLOWER BLOSSOMS

This movement exercises the whole body with a full skeletal stretch. It increases the elasticity of skin and muscles, and also releases tension. This movement follows on from Raindrops Fall on Lotus.

Movement breakdown

Movements

1. Unfold fists as you roll palms to face upwards, fingertips pointing towards the head.
2. Raise the body by straightening the knees. At the same time push hands over the head, palms facing up. Once legs are straight, push upwards on the balls of the feet, raising the heels only so far as is comfortable (in order to maintain balance).

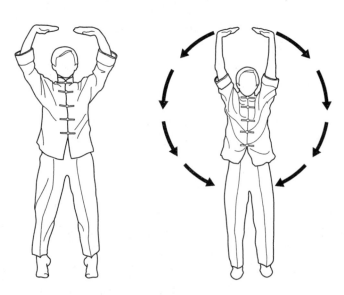

3. Lower heels gently to the ground and bend knees slightly. At the same time continue the outward arcing movement of the hands until they are brought downwards to the sides of the body.

Breathing

Breathe in as you raise the body and take the hands above the head. Breathe out as you lower the body and bring the hands down to the sides.

Mental imagery

Imagine you are a lotus flower which is opening.

Important points

- Do not over-extend the upward stretch so that you lose your balance and the correct posture.
- Keep neck relaxed and do not look upwards using the head.

FACE THE WIND

The waist and abdominal movements help the digestive and excretory functions. This movement also strengthens the internal organs and improves spinal mobility. It follows on from Lotus Flower Blossoms.

Movement breakdown

Movements

1. Turn right hand palm up, fingers pointing to the front.
2. Raise left hand to heart height, palm facing upwards, and roll wrist so that palm faces to the right, fingertips pointing upwards.
3. Roll wrist of right hand so palm faces downwards. At the same time turn waist 90 degrees to the right, raising the body by straightening the legs slightly.
4. Gently push left palm outwards to the right. Feel the stretch.
5. Gently push right palm downwards. At the same time lower the body by bending the knees slightly.

Roll left wrist to turn palm upwards, then slowly turn the body back 90 degrees to the central position and relax left hand in towards the hips. The left arm is now by the left side of the body.

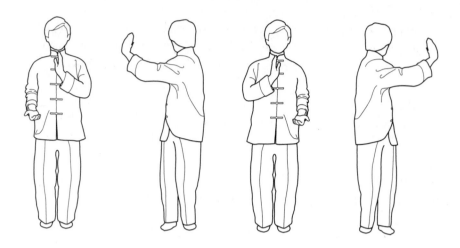

The above movements are now repeated on the other side of the body:
1. Turn left hand palm up, fingers pointing to the front.
2. Raise right hand to heart height, palm facing upwards. At the same time roll wrist so that palm faces to the left, fingertips pointing upwards.
3. Roll wrist of left hand so palm faces downwards. At the same time turn waist 90 degrees to the left, raising the body by straightening the legs slightly.
4. Gently push right palm outwards to the left. Feel the stretch.
5. Gently push left palm downwards. At the same time lower the body by bending the knees slightly.
6. Roll right wrist to turn palm upwards, then slowly turn the body back 90 degrees to the central position and relax right hand in towards the hips. The right arm is now by the right side of the body.

Breathing
Breathe in during the preparatory hand movements.
Breathe out as you raise the body and press to the right.
Breathe in during the second lot of preparatory hand movements.
Breathe out as you raise the body and press to the left.

Mental imagery
Imagine you are pressing your hand against the wind. Try to feel a strong, cool breeze blowing against the palm; feel as though you have to push against it.

Important points

- Keep head and spine erect; do not lean as you turn.
- Do not turn so far that you twist the knees; the turning is done in the waist.

LIFT THE SKY, PRESS THE EARTH

This movement exercises the back, strengthens the abdominal muscles, and improves the digestive system. It should also lift the spirits. This movement follows on from Face the Wind.

Movement breakdown

Movements
1. Place the left hand in the right palm, palms facing up, about navel height.
2. Raise the body by straightening the legs. At the same time lift hands up to chest height.
3. Keeping the left hand in the right palm, turn palms to face downwards.
4. Bending from the waist, push hands downwards towards the floor.
5. Bend knees as far as is comfortable.
6. While slowly bringing the body back to a vertical position, separate the hands, arcing them outwards and backwards (palms facing outwards, fingers pointing away from the body) to about waist height, then relax both arms in towards the body.

Breathing
Breathe in as you raise the body and lift the hands up.
Breathe out as you bend forwards.
Breathe in as you bring the body back to a vertical position.

Mental imagery
Imagine lifting a heavy weight as you bring the hands up and pressing down into the ground as you push them downwards.

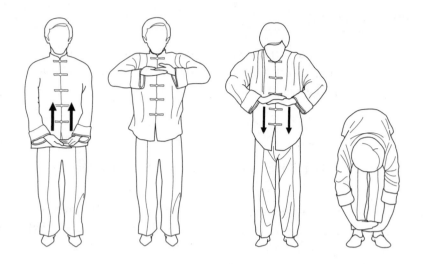

Important points

- Do not bend spine.
- Keep heels on the floor.
- Keep head in a straight line from the spine, eyes looking down; do not bend the neck to look upwards or forwards.
- Keep knees pointing to the front; do not turn them inwards to act as a brace for the body weight.

WHITE CRANE SPREADS WINGS

This movement exercises the wrists and arms, strengthens the abdominal muscles, and improves the excretory functions. It follows on from Lift the Sky, Press the Earth.

Movement breakdown

Movements

1. With fingertips leading, bring the hands to heart height, palms facing up.
2. By rolling wrists, turn right palm down and angle left palm outwards.
3. Raise the body by straightening the legs.
4. Push right palm downwards as far as possible, palm facing

downwards, fingertips pointing forwards. At the same time push left palm above the head as far as possible, palm facing upwards, fingertips pointing backwards (feeling the stretch), and lower the body by bending the knees slightly.

5. Relax the stretch and draw both hands back to heart height, as before, palms facing up.
6. By rolling the wrists, turn left palm down and angle right palm outwards.
7. Raise the body by straightening the legs.
8. Push left palm downwards as far as possible, palm facing downwards, fingertips pointing forwards. At the same time push right palm above the head as far as possible, palm facing upwards, fingertips pointing backwards (feeling the stretch).

Breathing

Breathe out as you bring the hands towards the heart, and raise the body. Breathe in as you stretch the hands downwards and upwards and raise the body.

Mental imagery

Imagine you are a white crane that has been hunting for fish and is now drying its wings in the sun, stretching them first one way and then another.

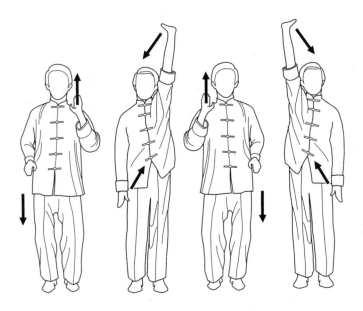

Important points

- Coordinate hand movements so that both hands reach heart height and the extension of the stretch at the same time.

SNOW RABBIT PLOUGHS THE EARTH

The benefits for this movement are the same as those for Snow Rabbit Digs the Earth. It follows on from White Crane Spreads Wings.

Movement breakdown

Movements

1. Lower the body by bending the knees slightly. At the same time draw the right hand down and bring the left hand up so that they meet in front of the centerline of the body, crossing at the wrists. Elbows are about chest height and the crossed hands are face height, with palms facing downwards, fingertips pointing at an upwards angle.

2. Keeping wrists crossed, arc hands downwards until palms come to face the body.

3. Continue the arcing movement, drawing hands up the center of the body. As the backs of the hands face forwards, separate hands so that arms are extended in front of the body at shoulder height, shoulder width apart. Palms face up and fingertips point to the front. Feel the stretch.

4. Raise the body by straightening the legs. At the same time relax the stretch and arc hands downwards slightly to the rear of the body, palms facing forwards and fingers downwards.

Breathing

Breathe out as you cross the hands and arc them downwards.
Breathe in as you bring the hands up in front of the body.
Breathe out as you separate the hands and bring them down.

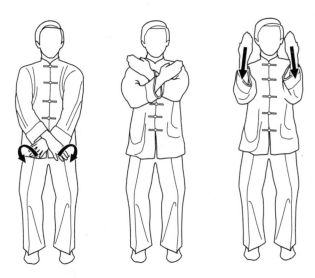

Mental imagery

Imagine you are a rabbit foraging on the banks of a stream in the early morning. As your hands roll forwards in Movement 3, feel yourself scooping through soft, moist earth.

Important points

* It is most important to keep shoulders relaxed throughout this movement. If this is difficult, lower the elbows.

WAVE HANDS IN AIR

This movement has the same benefits as Waving Hands. It follows on from Snow Rabbit Ploughs the Earth.

Movement breakdown

Movements

1. Lower the body by relaxing the knees. At the same time arc hands upwards and outwards to chest height, palms facing up and fingertips pointing towards the front. Feel the stretch.
2. Raise the body by straightening the legs. At the same time turn palms over to face downwards and press down to the sides of the body. Feel the stretch and then relax.
3. Lower the body with knees offlock.

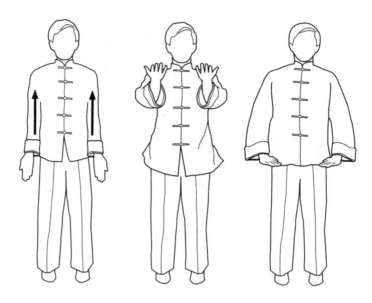

Breathing

Breathe in as you lower the body and raise the hands.

Breathe out as you raise the body and lower the hands.

Breathe in and then out as you lower the body at completion of the movement.

After completion of the final posture, take a minimum of three deep, calming breaths.

Mental imagery

Imagine the sun sinking below the horizon; the world becomes dark and quiet. Feel a sense of inner calmness and relaxation. Allow your eyes to close, and focus on your breathing while enjoying the sense of relaxation. When you are ready, slowly open your eyes without focusing; just let the light in. Then, again when you are ready, focus the eyes.

Important points

- Keep shoulders relaxed.

Bibliography

Cai, Jngeng, *Eating Your Way to Health — Dietotherapy in Traditional Chinese Medicine*, 2nd ed, Foreign Language Press, Beijing, 1996.

Jou, Tsung Hwa, *The Tao of Tai Chi Chuan — Way to Rejuvenation*, Charles E. Tuttle Co., Rutland, Vermont, 1980.

Khor, Gary, *Tai Chi Qigong — For Stress Control and Relaxation*, Simon & Schuster Australia, Sydney, 1993.

Liu, Zhengcai, *The Mystery of Longevity*, Foreign Language Press, Beijing, 1990.

Reid, Daniel, *The Tao of Health, Sex and Longevity*, Simon & Schuster, London, 1989.

Veith, Ilsa, *The Yellow Emperor's Classic of Internal Medicine*, University of California Press, Berkeley, 1972.

Index